Guided Surgery in Implantology

Kristian Kniha · Karl Andreas Schlegel
Heinz Kniha

Guided Surgery in Implantology

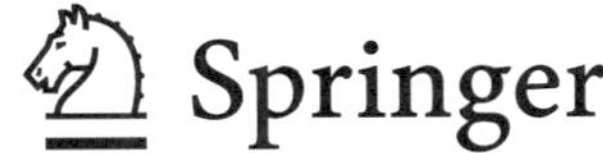

Springer

Kristian Kniha
Department of Oral and
Cranio-Maxillofacial Surgery
University Hospital RWTH
Aachen
Germany

Heinz Kniha
Kniha, Schlegel and Colleagues
Private Clinic for Oral and Maxillofacial
Surgery
Munich
Germany

Karl Andreas Schlegel
Kniha, Schlegel and Colleagues
Private Clinic for Oral and Maxillofacial
Surgery
Munich
Germany

ISBN 978-3-030-75218-7   ISBN 978-3-030-75216-3   (eBook)
https://doi.org/10.1007/978-3-030-75216-3

This Springer imprint is published by the registered company Springer Nature Switzerland AG
The registered company address is: Gewerbestrasse 11, 6330 Cham, Switzerland

Preface

Dentists have always tried to develop and improve the individual therapy approach of their patients. Especially in the field of dental implantology, there has been intermittent development and improvement of treatment techniques, restoration concepts, and implant materials. Therefore, it is no surprise that the modern digitalization of various procedures has found its way in the field of implantology and patient care. In the following book, the editors intend to highlight all facets of computer-guided implantology. Dentists have the desire to provide their patients with the best possible care. Ideal planning, fast and minimally invasive implantation, and prosthodontic restoration are essential for an overall successful treatment. Today's digital possibilities not only allow exact planning but are also a great help in the ideal placement of each single implant body. This may lead to reduced surgery times and therefore favors an optimal treatment outcome. Not every patient reflects the same initial situation and may present individual challenges, also with regard to digital planning. In certain cases, full-guided surgery can bring great intraoperative advantages by precisely coding the implant position; however, in particular situations, the technique is currently reaching its limits. Consequently, this modern technique does not replace all surgical abilities in the field of dental implantology; nevertheless, it is a great tool of support. In the course of this book, you will learn the advantages and disadvantages of full-guided surgery, master technical challenges, and avoid initial sources of error. All techniques described are illustrated with numerous clinical images. You will be given reliable workflow protocols. Furthermore, we aim to provide an up-to-date overview of the literature and to define key points that are of great importance for the success of the treatment. This book addresses everyone who wants to get a deep insight into the current scientific background and the many possible clinical situations of guided implantology.

Aachen, Germany	Kristian Kniha
Munich, Germany	Karl Andreas Schlegel
Munich, Germany	Heinz Kniha

Acknowledgments

We would like to thank "Labor für Dentaltechnik Thomas Lassen GmbH (Starnberg, Germany)" for providing individual laboratory figures. The authors thank Dr. med. dent. Kim Clever (Private practice for maxillofacial surgery, Dr. med. Dr. med. dent. Korbinian Seyboth, Inningerstr. 2, Augsburg, Germany) for the excellent support with Chap. 5 and the literature review. Additionally, I would like to thank Univ.-Prof. Dr. med. Dr. med. dent. Frank Hölzle (Head & Chairman, Department of Oral and Maxillofacial Surgery, University Hospital of RWTH Aachen, Germany) for granting me the necessary time and support for this scientific work. Furthermore, the authors report no conflicts of interest related to this work.

Contents

Part I

Guided Surgery: A Step-by-Step Guide

Guided surgery includes the preoperative digital implant planning and subsequent precise surgical implementation of an implant insertion guided by a special template. In guided surgery, a diagnostic radiological scan is first performed to accurately assess the patient's oral status. The implants are positioned on the computer through various intermediate steps and stored in the form of a drilling template. This surgical drill guide is placed in the patient's mouth during the surgical procedure and can therefore provide incredibly high accuracy in placing dental implants, especially in the case of multiple implants and implants for fixed dentures or multiple bridges.

Benefits and Disadvantages of Guided Surgery (Flap vs. Flapless)

Learning Objective
- Do you know the pros and cons of digital implant planning?

In principle, guided surgery can be divided into two methods. It is important to compare dynamic template-guided with static template-guided implant surgery. Since dynamic-guided implant surgery is currently only applicable to a limited extent due to its more complicated handling and higher investment costs, this book concentrates exclusively on the mainly used static-guided implant surgery [1].

Furthermore, pilot-drill templates must be distinguished from full-guided templates.

Conventional drilling templates are also called "pilot-drill templates" and are used for the orientation of the surgeon. Often, these templates are either closed or vestibular opened for easier insertion of the pilot drill (Fig. 1.1a–c). During the production of the pilot-drill templates, the dental technician indicates the position that is most suitable from a prosthetic point of view. No hard-tissue analysis, such as matching radiological data files, is considered in this process.

These guides provide the surgeon with certain orientation. In addition, they are quick and easy to produce. If a conventional guide is planned, we recommend using the version of Fig. 1.1a without drilling sleeves. It should be noted that the bone situation has not yet been considered in the cast model planning. Using a guide without sleeves, the pilot drill can be placed individually according to the bone tissue. However, the authors do not recommend using the pilot-drill templates of Fig. 1.1b, c. This can quickly lead to an incorrect pilot drill as shown in the following example. In Fig. 1.2a–g, a clinical and radiographic situation of a missing premolar is presented. In this case, a conventional template was placed according to the adjacent and contralateral crowns (Fig. 1.2e). However, for correct implant positioning, the nearby roots have to be considered. In this example, the axes of the crown and root of the premolar in tooth position 34 showed a deviation and the conventional guide sleeve angled too close to the anterior root (Fig. 1.2f). Therefore, the surgeon had to correct the implant axis by hand, and the guide could only be used for punch marking (Fig. 1.2g). Alternatively, the incorrect positioning recorded in the X-ray image could be corrected by the technician. However, a new preoperative image would have to be taken, which is why the authors cannot recommend this procedure due to the higher radiation exposure and the workflow complexity.

When compared to pilot-drill templates, full-guided surgery enables prosthetically oriented implant backward planning and subsequent implant placement. During "backward planning," the treatment goal—in this case, optimal implant prosthetics—determines the therapy path. From this ideal implant-supported denture, planning is done "backward" in relation to the implant rest. (Fig. 1.3). The necessary measures to restore bone and soft tissue are included in the planning.

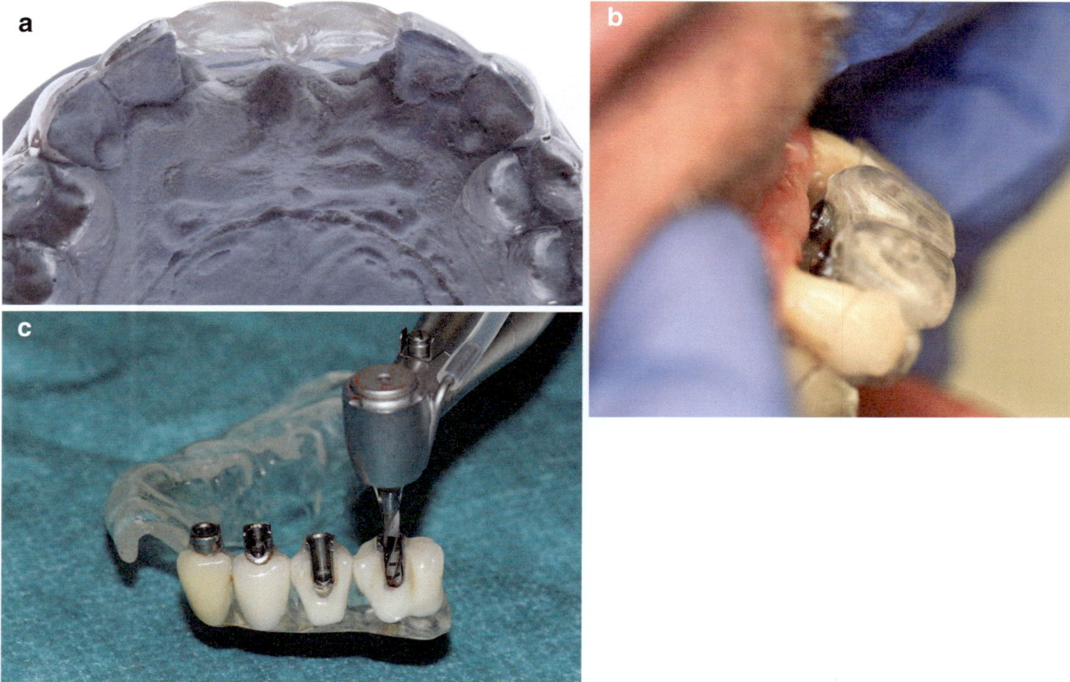

Fig. 1.1 (**a**) This template gives an orientation for either bone augmentation or subsequent implantation. In this case, the vestibular area of both missing central incisors represented the guiding help to which the bone augmentation and the implant axis can be aligned. (**b**) Conventional drilling template that is either closed or buccally opened for easier insertion of the drill. Only the pilot drill is guided by the template in this example. (**c**) Closed conventional drilling template guiding the pilot drill. (© Kristian Kniha 2021. All Rights Reserved)

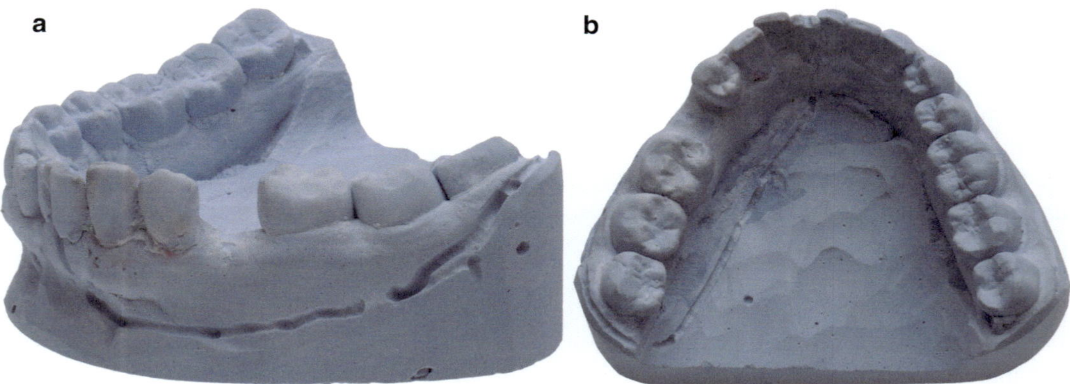

Fig. 1.2 (**a–d**) Example of a possible fabrication of a conventional guide. (**e**) When bringing together both cast models displaying the occlusion, the slightly backward inclined axis of the sleeve is visible. (**f, g**) After punch marking, the surgeon had to correct the implant axis by hand, and the template was not used for the pilot drill. (© Kristian Kniha 2021. All Rights Reserved)

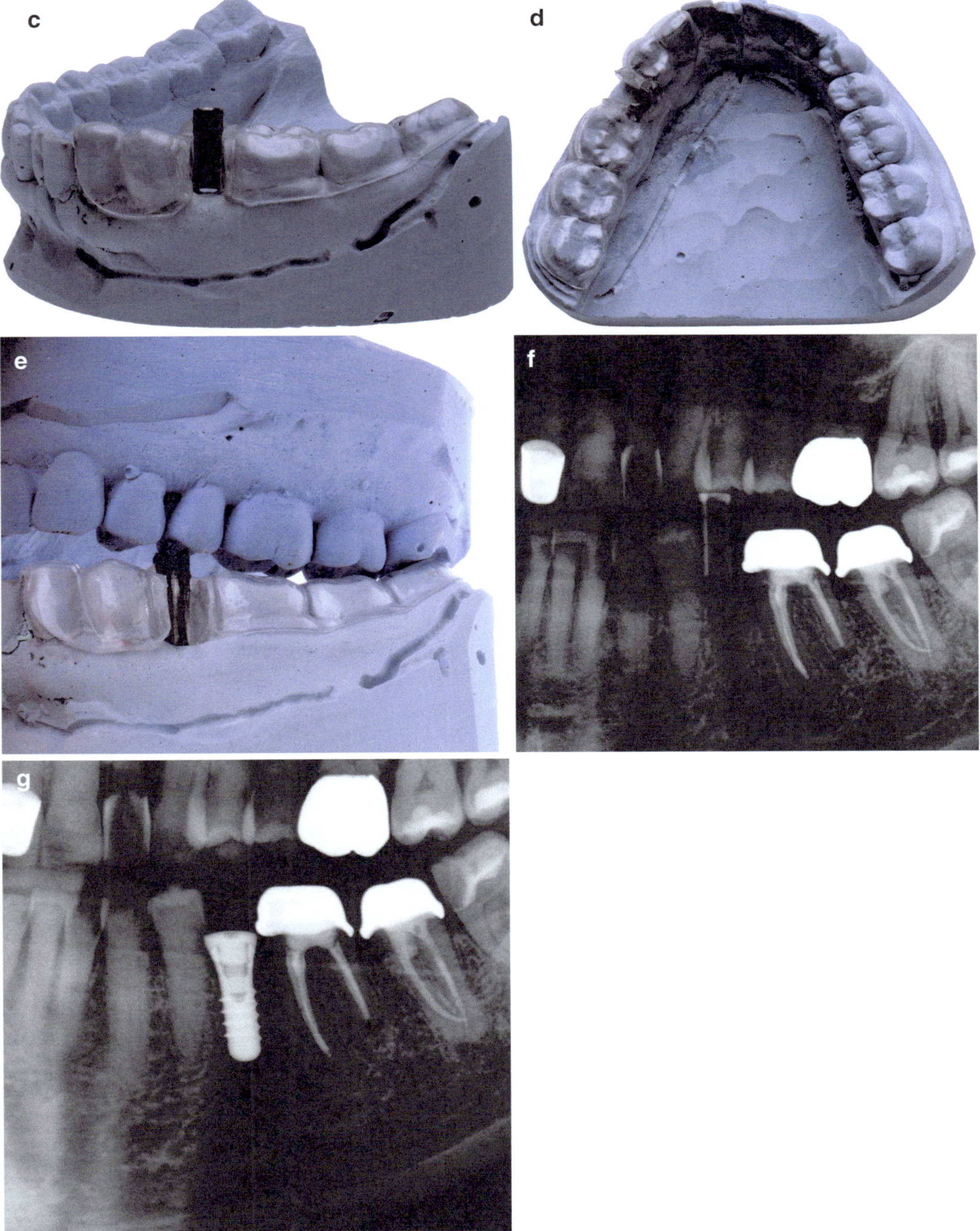

Fig. 1.2 (continued)

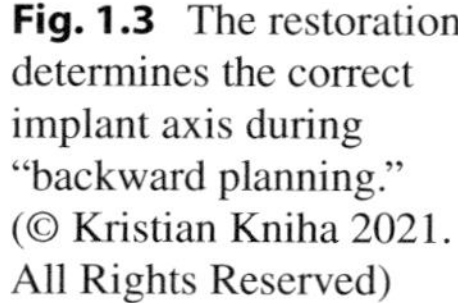

Fig. 1.3 The restoration determines the correct implant axis during "backward planning." (© Kristian Kniha 2021. All Rights Reserved)

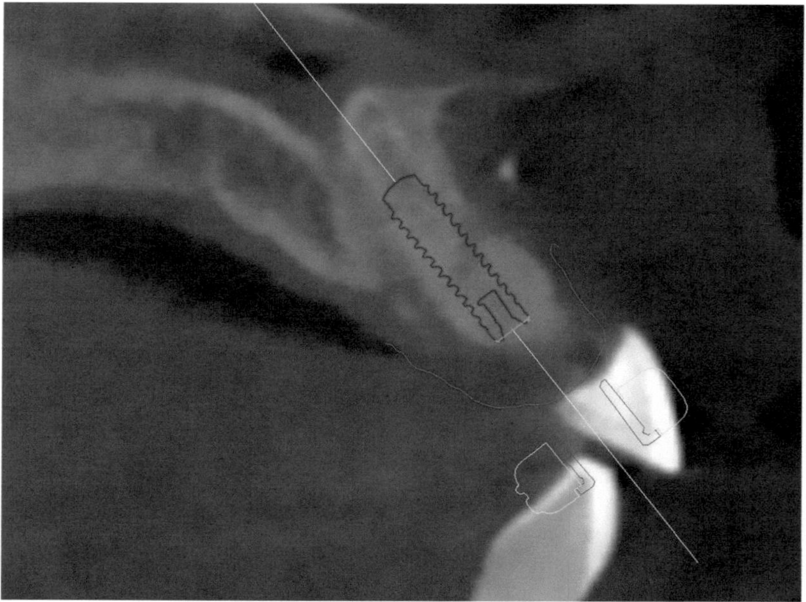

The treatment result is therefore predictable; any corrections are possible even before the actual surgical implantation.

Guided implantology uses three-dimensional radiological and clinical patient data in digital imaging and communications in medicine (DICOM) format to digitally examine, diagnose, and plan the treatment in order to put the planned surgery of the individual patient into practice [2].

Full-guided surgery usually consists of the following steps:

1. clinical preparation and medical imaging,
2. data collection and software planning,
3. fabrication of the guide,
4. full-guided implantation and, in selected cases, immediate prosthodontic restoration.

However, some variations in the workflow are possible and will be presented in Chap. 2.

Full-guided surgery allows for an exact, safe, and predictable planning [3, 4]. Additionally, the surgery time can be significantly reduced if the templates fit perfectly [2, 5].

According to the individual situation, within guided surgery, a flapless implant placement—which shortens the patient's healing time—may be performed more often [6]. This approach may avoid bone denudation (separation of bone and periosteum), maintaining a better vascular tissue supply, which might inhibit increased bone loss [6, 7]. Additionally, flapless surgery may keep gingiva profiles untouched, including the soft tissue margin position and interdental papillae [8]. However, not every full-guided surgery case should be planned with a flapless approach. According to Brodala's 2009 review, the surgical judgment of a flap vs. flapless approach for each case is related to the implant success rate [8]. The authors concluded that, on one hand, flapless surgery should not be performed on patients with a deficient initial soft tissue situation, such as reduced attached gingiva [4]. In the case of poor bony situations, creating a sufficient overview and gaining good access is crucial for closed healing by means of a flap preparation. Moreover, identifying the drilling depth in flapless surgery can be difficult, as there is no direct visualization of the bone [6].

Furthermore, flapless protocols prevent the opportunity for bone augmentations, such as an external sinus lift or a lateral bone graft. A wrong judgment in flapless vs. flap surgery may increase the risk of implant failure by up to 75% [9]. Nevertheless, full-guided surgery, a less invasive surgery with reduced bleeding and minimal postoperative pain for the patient, remains advantageous due to the exact preoperative planning and shorter surgery time [6]. Additionally, exact preoperative planning may allow immediate loading of the immediately inserted implants in special cases (Chap. 11) [4]. Thus, it is possible to already fabricate the provisional denture preoperatively, whereby the patient can leave the dental clinic directly with a temporary prosthesis.

The above-mentioned points emphasize the advantages of full-guided implantology. Some of the disadvantages, such as expensive investments, must also be mentioned. The preparation of three-dimensional data requires the commonly used cone-beam computer tomography (CBCT) or the even more expensive dental computer tomography (CT), which exposes the patient to higher doses of radiation compared to the CBCT [4]. If these X-ray devices are not available in the individual dental practice or clinic, the patient must be transferred to a radiological colleague initially. Variations can be observed in diagnostic image quality, showing substantial variability between CBCT technologies, exposure protocols, and subsequent analysis. In addition to the differences in image quality, the quality and quantity of the bone are also sometimes difficult to evaluate radiologically and may vary clinically [10]. Another major drawback is that the patient's distance of the incisal edges needs to be sufficient to accommodate the drills and templates for full-guided surgery. If the maximal distance of the incisal edges is less than 5 cm, the surgical procedure might not be possible, especially in the molar region [11]. A further disadvantage in planned flapless surgery, especially in initial difficult bony situations, consists of minimal and, therefore, insufficient access to the jaw bone [6]. Fortunately, a spontaneous switch from flapless access to surgery to a flap formation is usually possible but depends on the template design (Chap. 3). The change of strategy is borne at the expense of minimal invasiveness and extended surgery time. Another possible disadvantage is the increased time-consuming preoperative software planning. In the beginning, the surgeon and technician must become acquainted with the planning tools, resulting in an individual learning curve. Aside from that, full-guided surgery does not replace the necessary surgical skills

and experience, especially in difficult and unexpected intraoperative situations, such as a broken template or a major template inaccuracy noticed intraoperatively (Chap. 6).

Finally, using full-guided surgery involves additional costs for both practitioner and patient due to the initial purchase of expensive surgical kits [12] and the production costs of template fabrication by the dental technician plus the additional time consumed for planning.

1.1 Conclusion

Full-guided implantology holds numerous benefits, although each case should be reconsidered individually regarding the indications of guided surgery. According to the review of d'Haese et al., it can be concluded that no clear evidence suggesting that guided surgery is superior to conventional procedures in terms of treatment outcomes or efficiency yet exists [4]. Nevertheless, we recommended that inexperienced implantologists, in particular, use the support of full-guided surgery as often as possible.

References

1. Block MS, Emery RW, Cullum DR, Sheikh A. Implant placement is more accurate using dynamic navigation. J Oral Maxillofac Surg. 2017;75:1377–86.
2. Al YF, Camenisch B, Al-Sabbagh M. Is digital guided implant surgery accurate and reliable? Dent Clin N Am. 2019;63:381–97.
3. Bover-Ramos F, Vina-Almunia J, Cervera-Ballester J, Penarrocha-Diago M, Garcia-Mira B. Accuracy of implant placement with computer-guided surgery: a systematic review and meta-analysis comparing cadaver, clinical, and in vitro studies. Int J Oral Maxillofac Implants. 2018;33:101–15.
4. D'haese J, Ackhurst J, Wismeijer D, De Bruyn H, Tahmaseb A. Current state of the art of computer-guided implant surgery. Periodontology. 2017;2000(73):121–33.
5. Schwarz D, Kabbasch C, Scheer M, Mikolajczak S, Beutner D, Luers JC. Comparative analysis of sialendoscopy, sonography, and CBCT in the detection of sialolithiasis. Laryngoscope. 2015;125:1098–101.
6. Laverty DP, Buglass J, Patel A. Flapless dental implant surgery and use of cone beam computer tomography guided surgery. Br Dent J. 2018;224:601–11.

7. Staffileno H. Significant differences and advantages between the full thickness and split thickness flaps. J Periodontol. 1974;45:421–5.

8. Brodala N. Flapless surgery and its effect on dental implant outcomes. Int J Oral Maxillofac Implants. 2009;24(Suppl):118–25.

9. Chrcanovic BR, Albrektsson T, Wennerberg A. Flapless versus conventional flapped dental implant surgery: a meta-analysis. PLoS One. 2014;9:e100624.

10. Jacobs R, Salmon B, Codari M, Hassan B, Bornstein MM. Cone beam computed tomography in implant dentistry: recommendations for clinical use. BMC Oral Health. 2018;18:88.

11. Malo P, De Araujo Nobre M, Lopes A. The use of computer-guided flapless implant surgery and four implants placed in immediate function to support a fixed denture: preliminary results after a mean follow-up period of thirteen months. J Prosthet Dent. 2007;97:S26–34.

12. Pozzi A, Polizzi G, Moy PK. Guided surgery with tooth-supported templates for single missing teeth: a critical review. Eur J Oral Implantol. 2016;9(Suppl 1):S135–53.

Clinical Preparation for Guided Surgery and Medical Imaging (Different Workflows, Data Matching, and Segmentation)

Learning Objective

- Do you know which data sets have to be imported into the software and then superimposed for digital planning?

With the aid of computer-assisted planning, a full-guided template that provides precise guidance for all implant drills and implant insertion can be fabricated [1]. At first, a treatment plan should be created and each patient examined for critical anatomical structures. The treatment plan should include questions such as: What is the patient's wish in terms of removable or fixed denture, partially or completely edentulous situation, screw-retained crowns, telescopic or bar fixation of the removable prosthesis, and cemented or screw-retained fixed dentures? Is an augmentation necessary? One should also take into account the patient anamnesis and different loading protocols (immediate vs. delayed implant loading).

Using backward planning, the implants will be placed exactly according to the desired prosthetic position.

At first, the planned crown position should be determined within the framework of a wax-up. The wax-up can be performed either conventionally or digitally. In order to generate a diagnostic digital wax-up, three options are available (Table 2.1). Option number one is to transfer a conventional wax-up into an X-ray template. In option two, the superposition of the scanned wax-up STL files (Standard Triangle Language) is carried out in the planning software. Finally, a

Table 2.1 Available wax-up options

Transfer of a conventional wax-up into an X-ray template
Superposition of scanned wax-up STL files in the planning software
Digital wax-up directly in the planning software

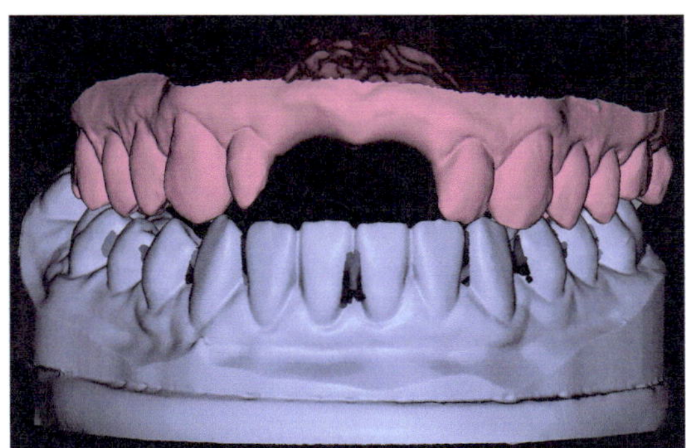

Fig. 2.1 Digital planning of the crown and implant positions in tooth positions 11 and 21. (© Karl Andreas Schlegel 2021. All Rights Reserved)

digital wax-up may be created directly in the planning software (Figs. 2.1 and 2.2).

Digital planning requires different data files that will be matched in the software. The CBCT data are exported in DICOM format. In the case of optical scans, such as scans of the cast model or oral scans, the STL format is mainly used. The software of the planning programs available on the market differs in structure and workflow. There are also numerous third-party implant

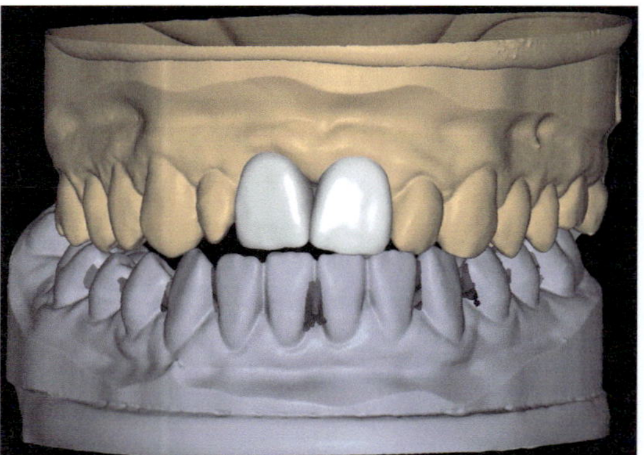

Fig. 2.2 The 3D wax-up was performed directly in the planning software (Exocad, BEGO GmbH, Bremen, Germany). (© Karl Andreas Schlegel 2021. All Rights Reserved)

Table 2.2 Available workflow options for data acquisition

Workflow I: X-ray template during CBCT scan
Workflow II: Software fusion
Workflow III: Double scan technique

planning software programs, such as SimPlant (Materialise Dental Inc., Glen Burnie, MD, USA), OnDemand3D (Cybermed Inc., Seoul, Korea), Virtual Implant Placement software (Bio-Horizons, Inc., Birmingham, AL, USA), Invivo5 (Anatomage, San Jose, CA, USA), NobelClinician (Nobel Biocare, Goteborg, Sweden), coDiagnostiX (Dental Wings Inc., Montreal, CA, USA), and Blue Sky Plan (BlueSkyBio, LLC, Grayslake, IL, USA) [2]. In Table 2.2, different workflows for data acquisition and matching are presented.

Some workflows require a radiopaque scan prosthesis with reference bodies to be placed in the mouth during the CBCT scan, while others do not.

2.1 Workflow I: X-ray Template During CBCT Scan

In workflow I, impressions of both jaws are taken to generate cast models with a wax-up at the planned implant positions (Figs. 2.3 and 2.4). Subsequently, the dental technician fabricates the radiopaque scan prosthesis based on a tooth setup (Fig. 2.4b) [2]. When the patient is scanned with the incorporated scan prosthesis in the CBCT, the desired tooth setup will be visible in the radiographic image and, therefore, in the planning software. This setup supplies the surgeon with the necessary prosthetic information for implant planning (Fig. 2.4c–e).

If the radiopaque scan prosthesis shows a perfect fit before and during the CBCT, an ideal fit during the following surgery can be expected. Furthermore, metal artifacts in the CBCT do not affect the fit of the template during surgery. However, the manufacturing process is more complex.

For the representation of the soft tissue lining, an STL file of the jaw can be imported and matched in the planning software. This STL file can be superimposed on the CBCT file using the maximum possible superposition adjusted by the automatic software function (Fig. 2.5a–c) [3]. In a semi-manual process, the surgeon should select at least three pairs of points for accurate matching. Thus, Fig. 2.5c now combines the information of the hard and soft tissue.

2.2 Workflow II: Software Fusion

For the process of software fusion, it is recommended to have at least 4–6 teeth in at least 2 quadrants to achieve a precise workflow [3]. First, impressions of each jaw and a CBCT scan without any radiographic template of the patient are required. If necessary, old CBCT scans may be used, provided the scan is not too old and does not show substantial differences from the current hard- and soft-tissue situation. However, we recommend starting with CBCT to get information about the bone situation at the beginning. The impression and possible wax-up information will then be sent to the technician. Subsequently, digital scans are made once with the plaster model and once with the wax-up with a laboratory scanner.

Alternatively, using a virtual diagnostic model, the diagnostic wax-up may also be performed using special software (Figs. 2.1 and 2.2). The option of creating a digital wax-up using the planning tool has the advantage that no dental technician is necessary [4]. This procedure is rather suitable for protocols with few single implants in partially edentulous patients [5].

Workflow I
X-ray template during CBCT scan

1. Clinical diagnostics and impressions of both jaws

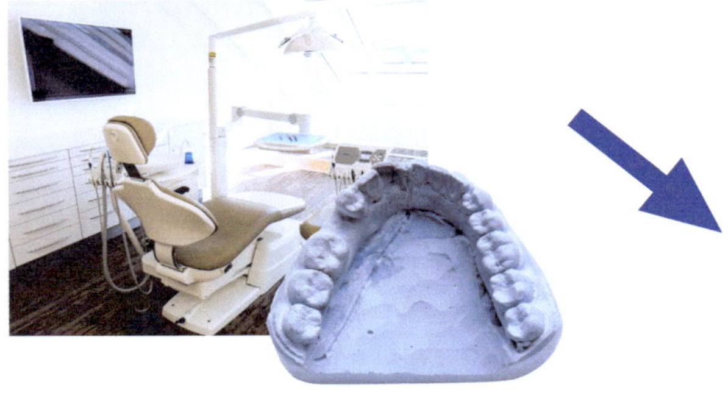

2. CBCT scan with a fabricated radiographic guide

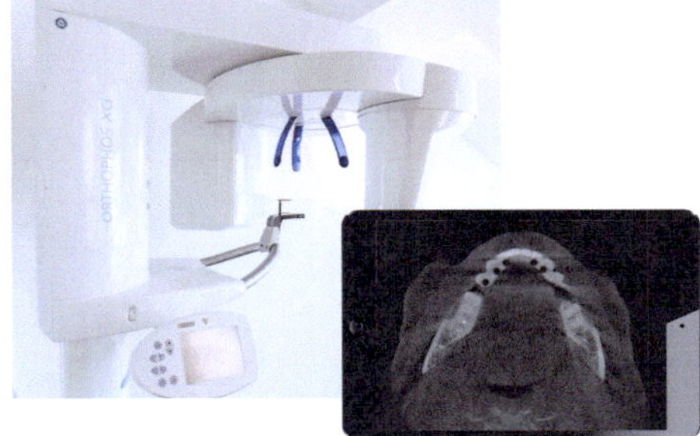

3. Treatment planning

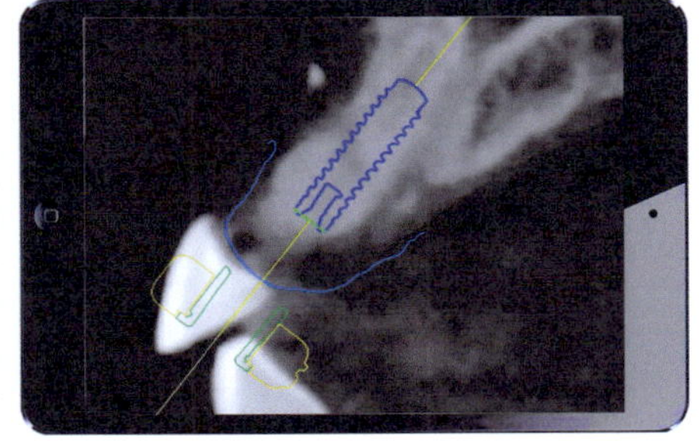

4. Guided surgery

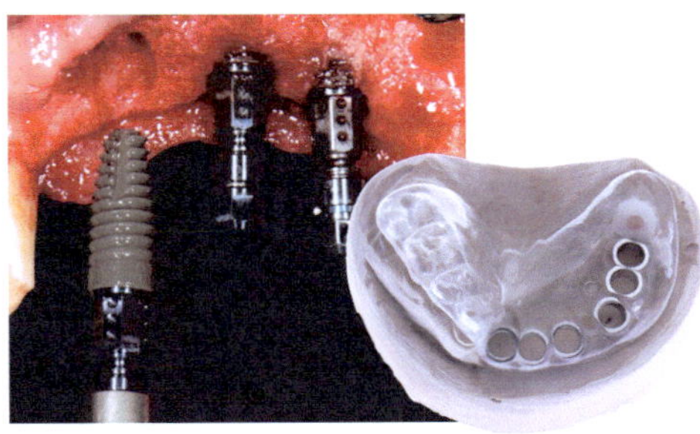

Fig. 2.3 Overview of workflow I. (© Kristian Kniha 2021. All Rights Reserved)

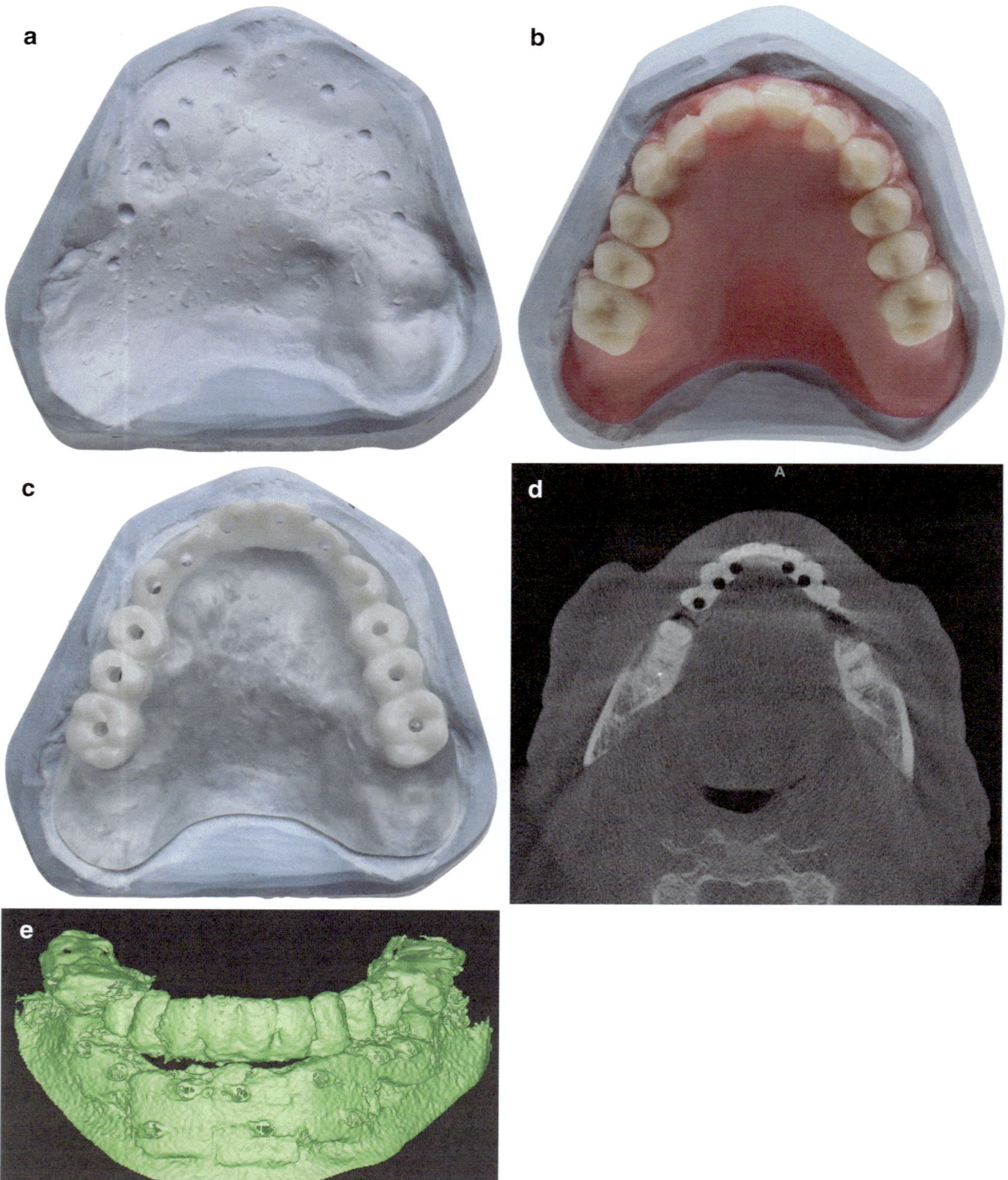

Fig. 2.4 (**a–c**) The radiopaque scan prosthesis based on a wax-up was fabricated and subsequently inserted during the CBCT scan. A duplicate of the old existing prosthesis can also be used as a wax-up. (**d**) The radiographic template is visible in the CBCT scan indicating the crown axis and position with holes (other case). (**e**) The tooth setup will therefore be transferred to the planning software. This image was taken after the segmentation process. (© Kristian Kniha 2021. All Rights Reserved)

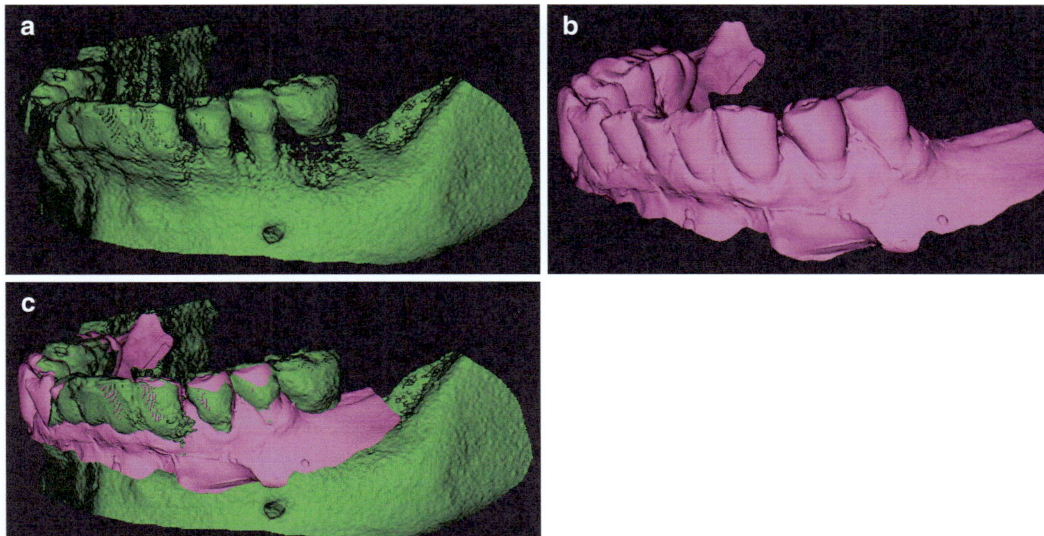

Fig. 2.5 (**a**) In this case, an implant was planned in position 36 and the patient was scanned with the incorporated scan prosthesis in the CBCT. The green area represents hard tissue. (**b**) This image shows the scan of the model cast (pink) of the lower jaw. (**c**) Both files were superimposed in the planning software (coDiagnostiX, Dental Wings Inc., Montreal, CA, USA). On the other hand, using the software fusion in workflow II, a cast model with temporary dentures or a wax-up can be scanned with a model scanner, or an optical impression can be used for the information of the individual tooth setup (Fig. 2.6). Avoiding the X-ray templates of the workflow I will result in considerable time and cost savings for the patient. (© Kristian Kniha 2021. All Rights Reserved)

The two resulting STL files are then sent back to the surgeon. Now, the CBCT and the laboratory images are matched together. Usually, well-defined tooth areas should be selected on both sides. Once the alignment is complete, implant planning can begin [3].

2.3 Workflow III: Double Scan Technique

The double-scan technique uses two CBCT scans, one with the integrated X-ray template and one with the template itself (Fig. 2.7).

The density of the radiographic template and surrounding soft tissue are indistinguishable and therefore impossible to segment from CBCT images [3]. With this technique, either the prosthesis or the radiographic template uses markers for later alignment. Consequently, the registration marks on the template were scanned once in the patient's mouth, followed by a second scan of the template itself. Various options are described in the literature for overlaying intraoral scans and CBCT data. For example, Flügge et al. matched the teeth, Dolcini et al., Oh et al., and An et al. placed radiopaque markers (e.g., gutta-percha or radiopaque composite) on the denture, teeth, or gingiva [6–9]. The radiographic markers allow these two scans to be matched together to show the position of the denture in relation to the underlying hard and soft tissue (Fig. 2.8a, b). In the protocol of the radiographic template, an impression of both jaws is required to make a wax-up and to fabricate the template. A bite index is required to ensure the correct position of the template or denture. Once the matching is complete, the software allows the clinician to begin implant planning based on the anatomical and prosthetic data.

Workflow II
Software fusion

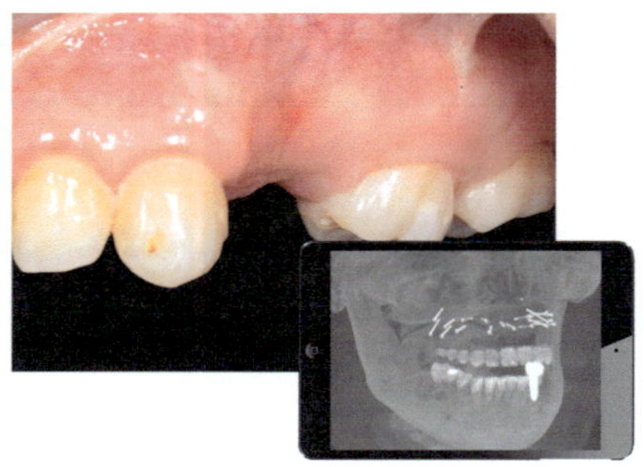
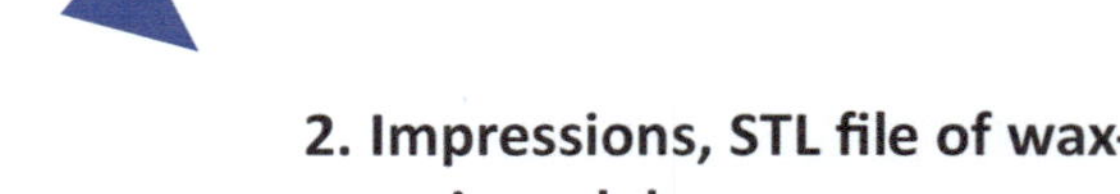

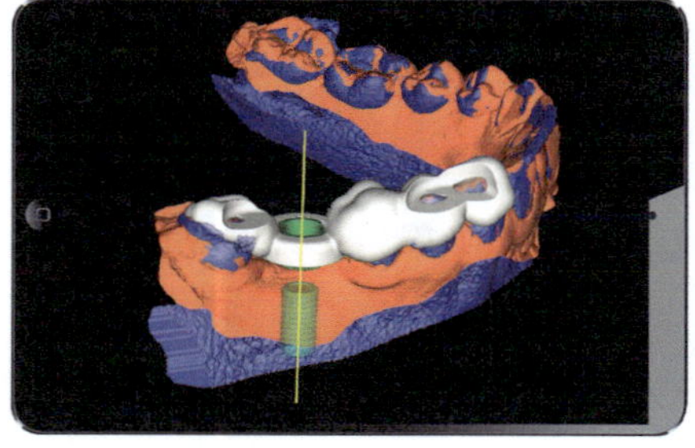

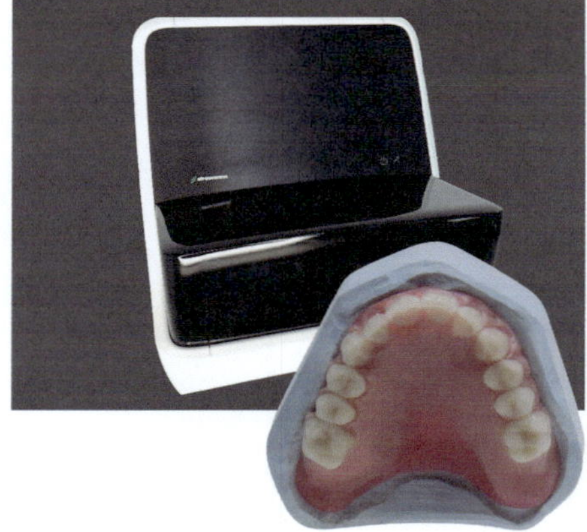
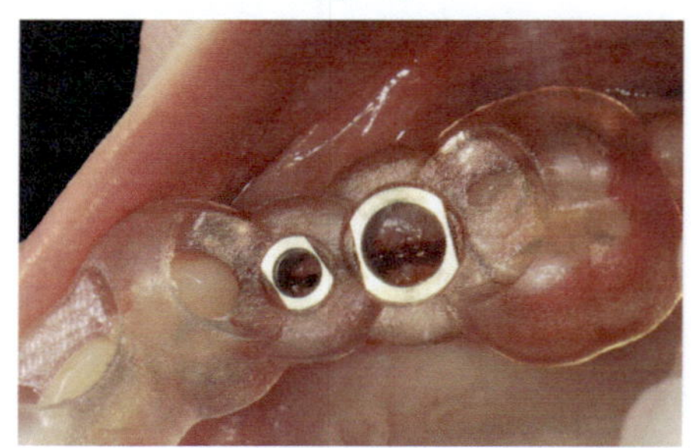

Fig. 2.6 Overview of workflow II. (© Kristian Kniha 2021. All Rights Reserved)

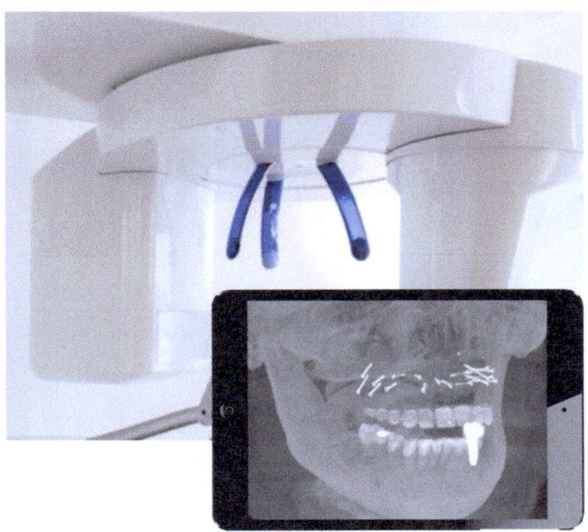

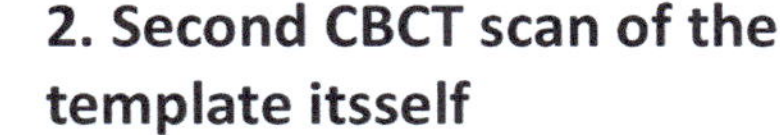

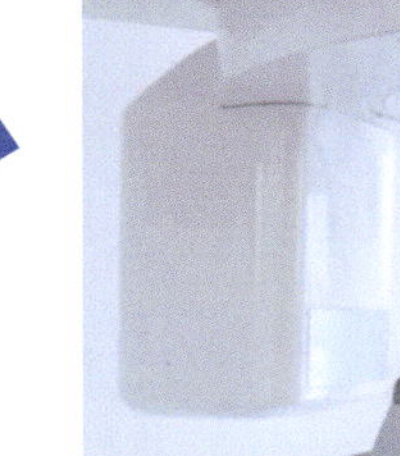

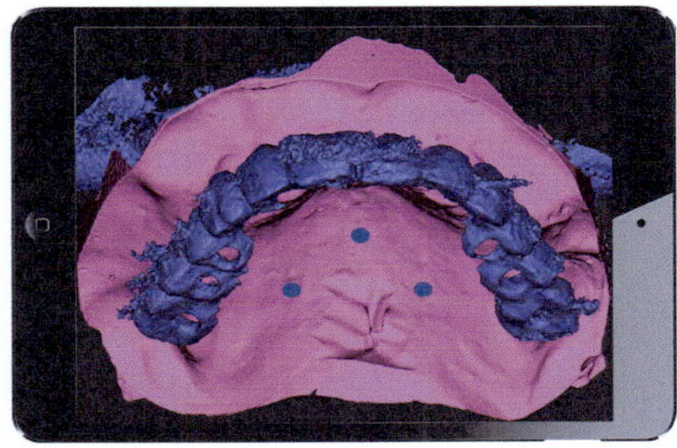

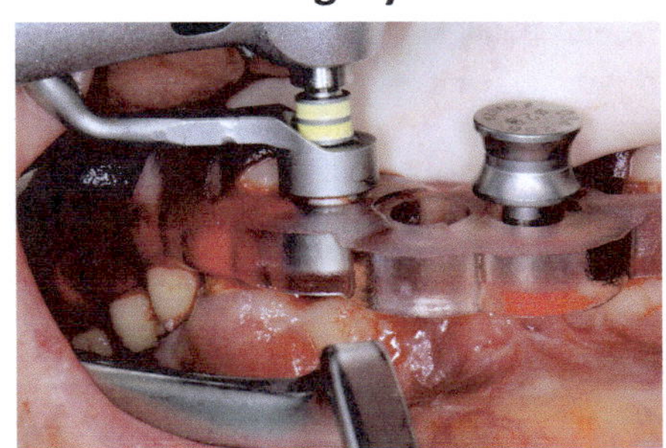

Fig. 2.7 Overview of workflow III. (© Kristian Kniha 2021. All Rights Reserved)

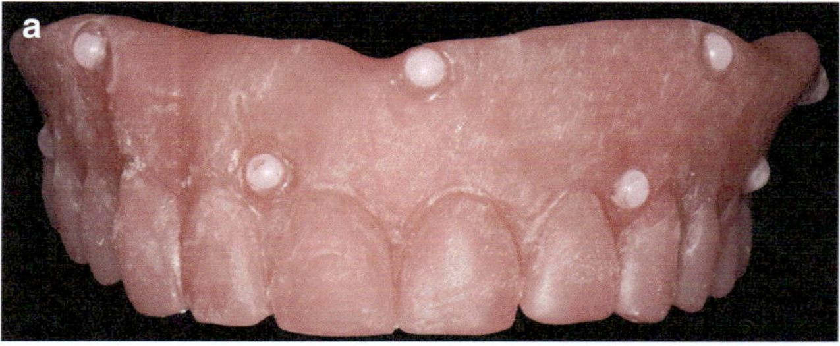
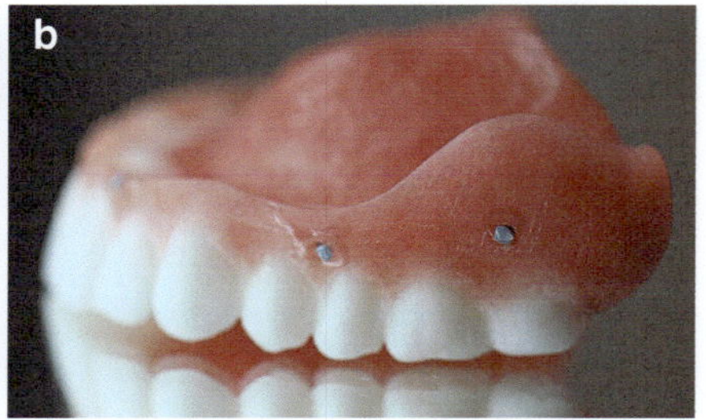

Fig. 2.8 (**a**) Reference notches were placed at the vestibular side of the template. The markers require a geometrical shape to produce a fixed and identifiable outline. (**b**) Radiopaque markers were bonded to the polished surface of the prosthesis on both sides. The radiopaque markers are embedded in the prosthesis and are identifiable in the CBCT images. (© Karl Andreas Schlegel 2021. All Rights Reserved)

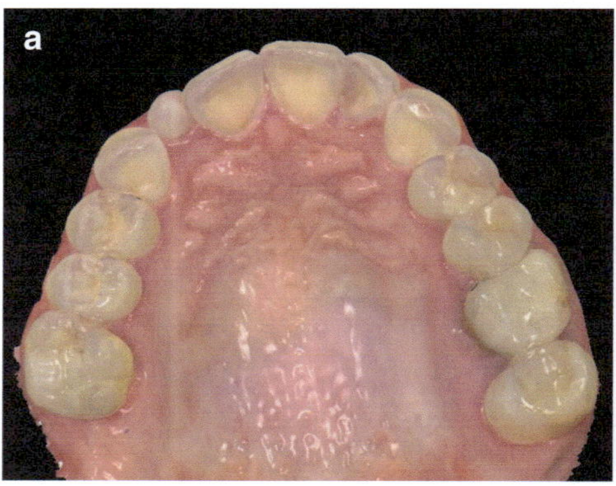
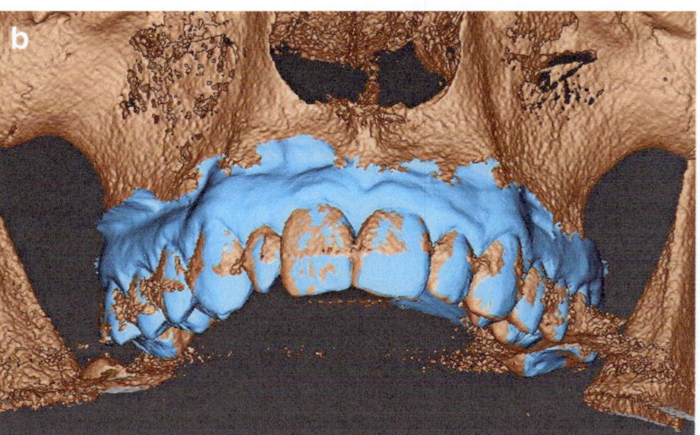

Fig. 2.9 (**a**) Optical impression of the upper jaw using the intraoral scanner by 3shape (Trios, 3Shape, Copenhagen, Denmark). (**b**) The digital information of the dento-gingival soft tissue and 3D data collected on the bony structure were superimposed within the implant planning software. (© Kristian Kniha 2021. All Rights Reserved)

2.4 Conventional or Digital Impressions

Impressions may be carried out conventionally or digitally. For example, a conventional impression uses alginate or polyvinyl siloxane and polyether. Afterward, the cast model with or without wax-up is digitalized with a cast model scanner, whereas a digital impression may be carried out using an intraoral scanner. Based on the computer-aided design/computer-aided milling (CAD/CAM) process, a cast model replica can be fabricated for the wax-up. Similarly, the wax-up on the replicated model will be digitalized with a cast model scanner. Optical impressions have several advantages over conventional impressions: they reduce discomfort for the patient, they are time-saving, and they eliminate the need for plaster casts (Fig. 2.9a, b) [10]. In addition to the individual optical scans of the upper and lower jaws, the occlusion is registered with the buccal scan.

Since the accuracy of optical impressions is similar to or better than that of alginate impressions, it can be assumed that the optical impression is recommended for diagnostic purposes [11]. Overall, there is still a tendency in the literature to favor polyvinyl siloxane and polyether impressions over optical ones [11]. However, this observation seems to depend on the extension of the impression. As the extension increases to cover the entire arch, the inferiority of the optical impressions becomes more apparent [11, 12]. Different timings of oral scans and their benefits are presented in Table 2.3.

Table 2.3 Advantages and disadvantages of the timing of the oral scan for the fabrication of the denture [13]

Timing of oral scan for implant loading	Denture	Indication	Predictable precision
Oral scan before implantation	• Temporary	• Immediate loading during surgery	• Limited • Less appointments
Oral scan during surgery	• Temporary or final	• Immediate loading or delayed loading at exposure	• Definite implant position • Reduced soft tissue predictability
Scan after the implant placement (e.g., exposure)	• Temporary or final	• Delayed loading	• Definite implant position • Most appointments • High soft tissue predictability

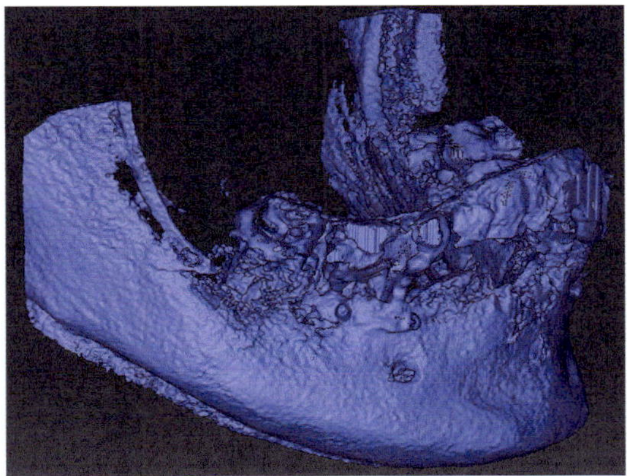

Fig. 2.10 This image shows possible metallic artifacts produced by crowns and implants in the CBCT scan, which may affect the matching accuracy. (© Kristian Kniha 2021. All Rights Reserved)

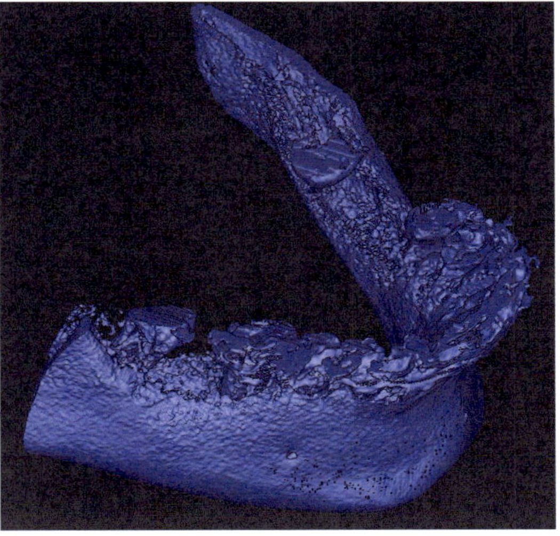

Fig. 2.11 Overlapping of the teeth will lead to missing parts of the crown after the segmentation process. (© Kristian Kniha 2021. All Rights Reserved)

In addition to impressions, radiological 3D scans are also necessary. Regardless of the imaging technology used, radiographic scanning with the correct parameters is the basis for optimal image quality and, therefore, for precise planning and correct implant placement. A systematic review assessed CBCT performance in terms of radiation doses and image quality [14]. Differences were observed in diagnostic image quality, showing substantial variability between CBCT technologies and exposure protocols. The diagnostic image quality can also be affected by patient factors, such as movement, and metal artifacts (Fig. 2.10).

During the scan, the patient's teeth should not be in contact. We recommend that the patients bite on cotton wool rolls to avoid overlapping. In this way, the complete occlusal surfaces can be used for matching afterward (Fig. 2.11).

With pre-implantological three-dimensional imaging and the use of an X-ray template, it must be ensured that there is a sufficient fit of the guide either on the remaining teeth or on the gingiva. If necessary, temporary mini-implants, for example, maybe used in edentulous jaws, as otherwise incorrect repositioning of the drilling template will lead to inaccuracies during surgery (Fig. 2.12).

Additionally, further standardization is needed for the grayscale output to be able to assess bone healing and condition [15].

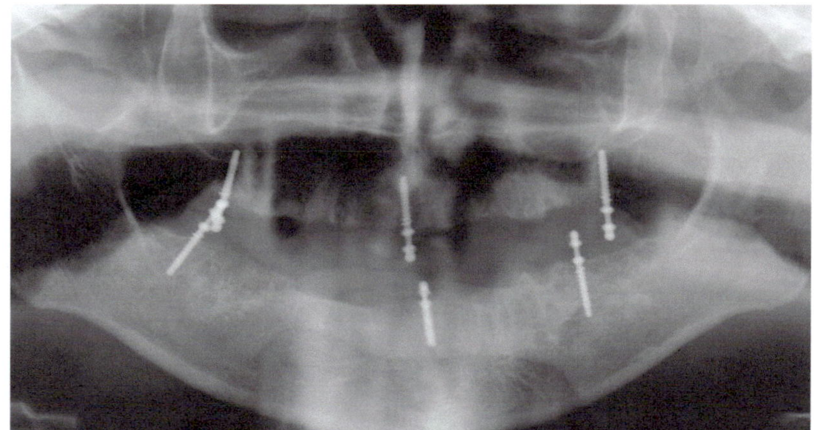

Fig. 2.12 In this case, due to the movable gingiva, mini-implants were used for correct template positioning. (© Karl Andreas Schlegel 2021. All Rights Reserved)

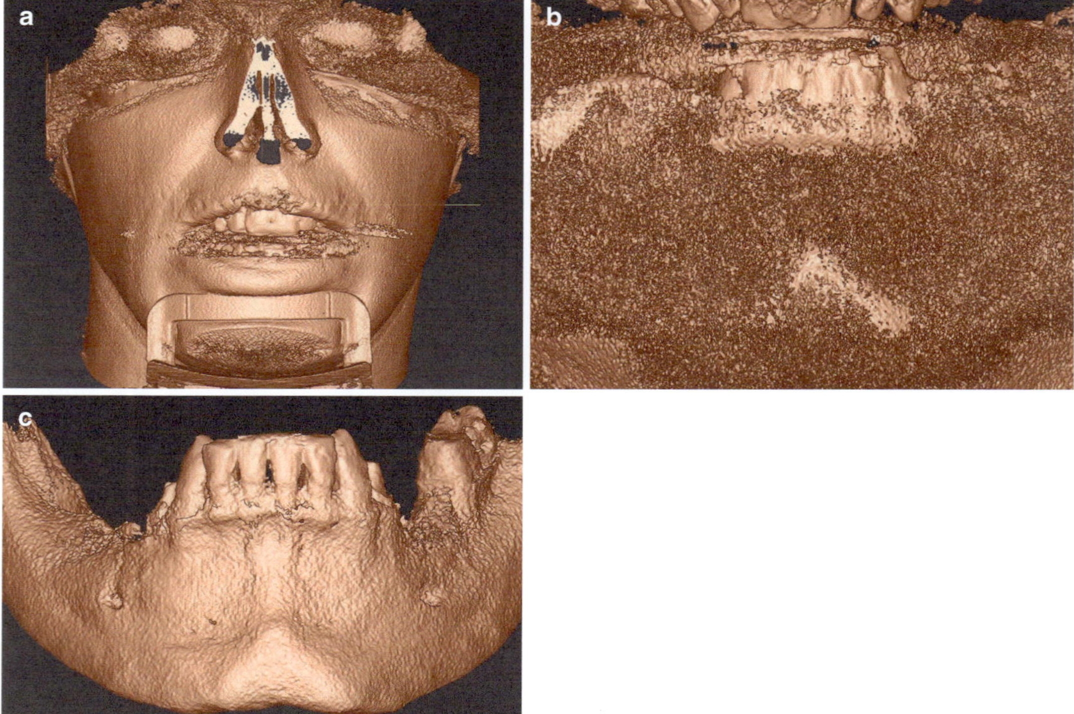

Fig. 2.13 (**a**) Initial CBCT import into the individual program for segmentation. (**b**) Calibrating the gray values will make tooth and jaw structures appear. (**c**) This example shows a fully segmented mandible. The crowns and the bony structures are clearly visible. It is recommended to work on each jaw separately. (© Kristian Kniha 2021. All Rights Reserved)

After the 3D scan, the DICOM data should be imported into the planning software. The next step consists of carrying out a so-called segmentation. Since the relevant information in the medical image should be most effectively presented to the surgeon, the raw data set is post-processed during segmentation: the radiological gray values have to be calibrated and the artifacts reduced (Fig. 2.13a, b). The segmentation should lead to correctly identifying common structures, such as teeth or jaw formations (Fig. 2.13c).

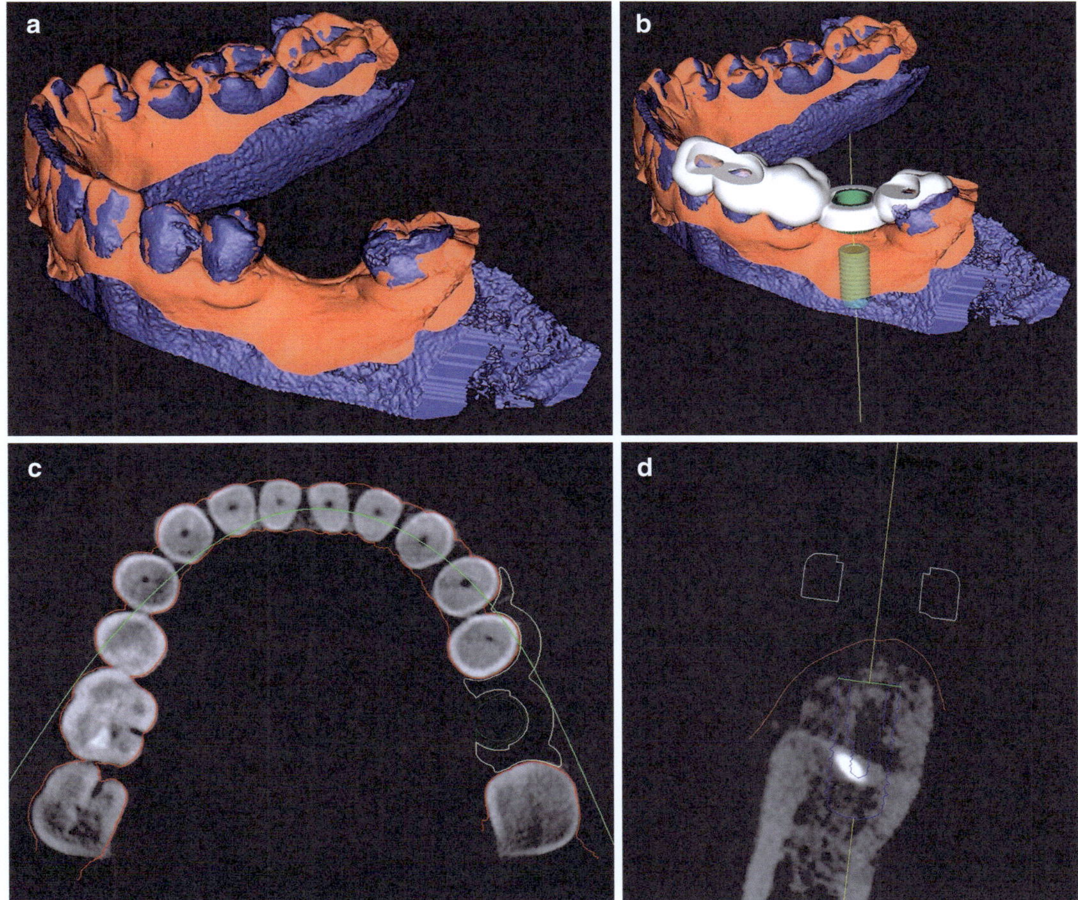

Fig. 2.14 (**a**) The matching accuracy of the model scan data with the CBCT data is sufficiently accurate for the remaining teeth. (**b**) Tooth-borne guides show the most accurate fit and support. (**c**) Axial view of the perfect matching accuracy between the model scan data and the crowns of the CBCT. (**d**) In this case, due to a sufficient bone volume, the implant is placed in 3D according to the backward planning of the crown position. (© Kristian Kniha 2021. All Rights Reserved)

The manual segmentation of 3D models by the surgeon proved to be significantly better than automatic segmentation, especially for patients with several metallic restorations leading to artifacts [16].

Depending on the planning protocol of the individual manufacturers, such as coDiagnostiX™ (Dental Wings, Chemnitz) and Galileos Implant (Sicat, Bonn), the data of the models/scans can be matched with the 3D image in the implant planning software. In some software programs, it is also possible to set up a diagnostic virtual tooth setup (Fig. 2.2) [13]. Clinical scans or scans of cast models may be imported into the software in order to match with visible references (Fig. 2.14a). With ≥4 remaining immobile teeth, the matching accuracy of the model scan data with the CBCT data is sufficiently accurate for implant planning and template-guided implementation (Fig. 2.14b, c) [15]. The automatic software function uses the maximum possible superposition of the clinical and radiographic situation in these cases (Fig. 2.14c, d).

However, in edentulous patients, due to missing distinctive matching references, inaccuracies may occur and must therefore be controlled and manually corrected. Often, the palate in the upper jaw provides sufficient reference for the matching accuracy (Fig. 2.15).

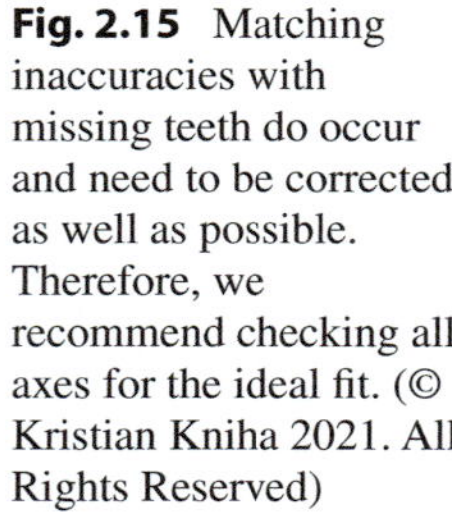

Fig. 2.15 Matching inaccuracies with missing teeth do occur and need to be corrected as well as possible. Therefore, we recommend checking all axes for the ideal fit. (© Kristian Kniha 2021. All Rights Reserved)

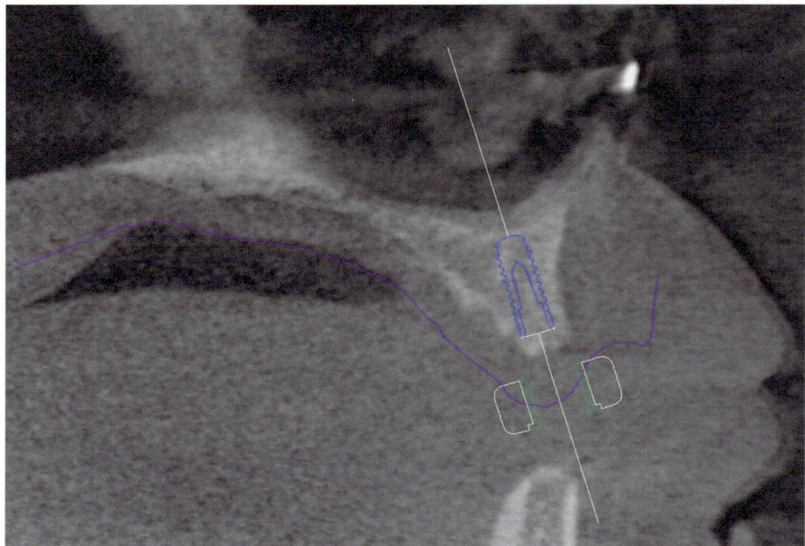

After achieving the segmentation and matching of all files, one can proceed with the next steps of implant planning. Full-guided surgery allows for implants to be placed virtually within the planning software. The three-dimensional representation of the bone, gingiva, and crown positions allows an exact implant placement.

2.5   Conclusion

Full-guided templates provide precise guidance for the implant drills and implant itself during insertion. As the extension increases to cover the entire arch, the inferiority of optical vs. conventional impressions becomes more apparent. Radiographic exposure protocols affect the diagnostic image quality. The segmentation and matching of files are necessary in order to proceed to the implant placement.

References

1. D'haese J, Van De Velde T, Komiyama A, Hultin M, De Bruyn H. Accuracy and complications using computer-designed stereolithographic surgical guides for oral rehabilitation by means of dental implants: a review of the literature. Clin Implant Dent Relat Res. 2012;14:321–35.
2. Mora MA, Chenin DL, Arce RM. Software tools and surgical guides in dental-implant-guided surgery. Dent Clin N Am. 2014;58:597–626.
3. Arcuri L, De Vico G, Ottria L, Condo R, Cerroni L, Mancini M, Barlattani A. Smart fusion vs. double scan: a comparison between two data-matching protocols for a computer guided implant planning. Clin Ter. 2016;167:55–62.
4. Stapleton BM, Lin WS, Ntounis A, Harris BT, Morton D. Application of digital diagnostic impression, virtual planning, and computer-guided implant surgery for a CAD/CAM-fabricated, implant-supported fixed dental prosthesis: a clinical report. J Prosthet Dent. 2014;112:402–8.
5. Happe A, Fehmer V, Herklotz I, Nickenig HJ, Sailer I. Possibilities and limitations of computer-assisted implant planning and guided surgery in the anterior region. Int J Comput Dent. 2018;21:147–62.
6. Flugge TV, Nelson K, Schmelzeisen R, Metzger MC. Three-dimensional plotting and printing of an implant drilling guide: simplifying guided implant surgery. J Oral Maxillofac Surg. 2013;71:1340–6.
7. Dolcini GA, Colombo M, Mangano C. From guided surgery to final prosthesis with a fully digital procedure: a prospective clinical study on 15 partially edentulous patients. Int J Dent. 2016;2016:7358423.
8. Oh JH, An X, Jeong SM, Choi BH. Digital workflow for computer-guided implant surgery in edentulous patients: a case report. J Oral Maxillofac Surg. 2017;75:2541–9.
9. An X, Yang HW, Choi BH. Digital workflow for computer-guided implant surgery in edentulous patients with an intraoral scanner and old complete denture. J Prosthodont. 2019;28:715–8.
10. Mangano F, Gandolfi A, Luongo G, Logozzo S. Intraoral scanners in dentistry: a review of the current literature. BMC Oral Health. 2017;17:149.

11. Abduo J, Elseyoufi M. Accuracy of intraoral scanners: a systematic review of influencing factors. Eur J Prosthodont Restor Dent. 2018;26:101–21.

12. Rutkunas V, Geciauskaite A, Jegelevicius D, Vaitiekunas M. Accuracy of digital implant impressions with intraoral scanners. A systematic review. Eur J Oral Implantol. 2017;10(Suppl 1):101–20.

13. Im J, Cha JY, Lee KJ, Yu HS, Hwang CJ. Comparison of virtual and manual tooth setups with digital and plaster models in extraction cases. Am J Orthod Dentofac Orthop. 2014;145:434–42.

14. Jacobs R, Salmon B, Codari M, Hassan B, Bornstein MM. Cone beam computed tomography in implant dentistry: recommendations for clinical use. BMC Oral Health. 2018;18:88.

15. Schnutenhaus S, Groller S, Luthardt RG, Rudolph H. Accuracy of the match between cone beam computed tomography and model scan data in template-guided implant planning: a prospective controlled clinical study. Clin Implant Dent Relat Res. 2018;20:541–9.

16. Flugge T, Derksen W, Te Poel J, Hassan B, Nelson K, Wismeijer D. Registration of cone beam computed tomography data and intraoral surface scans – A prerequisite for guided implant surgery with CAD/CAM drilling guides. Clin Oral Implants Res. 2017;28(9):1113–1118.

3

Preoperative Planning for Guided Surgery (Implant Positioning and Template Designs)

Learning Objective

- Are you aware of the ideal implant position in relation to the hard and soft tissue?

Guided surgery improves the visualization of the prosthetic outcome and transfer of the planned implant positions to the clinical situation [1]. The three-dimensional representation of the bone height and width makes it clear if and to what extent simultaneous augmentations are required.

After segmentation and superimposition with cast models if necessary, each implant can be imported and placed in the correct 3D position according to the hard and soft tissue and the correct prosthodontic crown position. Depending on the planning, a suitable implant type, position, diameter, and length can be selected.

According to the current literature, there are several studies that showed the perfect implant position in single gaps or in cases with adjacent implants. A distance of 1.5 mm between the implant and the neighboring teeth should always be kept in the mesiodistal position [2]. In Fig. 3.1a, a single premolar gap is presented. If possible, this position may be replaced with a regular neck (RN) implant (appr. 4 mm diameter). In the case of a narrowed tooth space, a narrow neck (NN) implant may be used.

When replacing a molar, it may be necessary to use an implant with a greater width in order to generate a harmonious profile between the implant shoulder and the crown (Fig. 3.1b). Additionally, with this approach, the distance between implants and the neighboring teeth should be kept at 1.5 mm. In the case of a narrowed tooth space, a regular implant may be used.

It has been shown that the interdental horizontal implant distance around titanium implants determines soft tissue behavior [3–5]. However, there is still no agreement on the ideal distance. While on the one hand, implant spacings of 1, 2, and 3 mm did not have a significant influence on the papilla height [6–8], on the other hand, there is a desire to maintain a minimum spacing of 3 mm or more [2, 5, 9, 10]. This is because smaller distances have often been associated with inter-implant bone loss and a missing papilla [3]. Therefore, there seems to be no general recommendation so far, although interdental distances of 3 mm around implants are more often associated with full papilla formation [3]. We recommend a horizontal distance of 2–3 mm between two implants (Fig. 3.1c). This distance may increase for adjacent implants in the molar position (appr. 3–4 mm) and may decrease for mandibular incisors (appr. 2 mm).

Buser et al. described the comfort zone in the esthetic zone: the implant should emerge at 1.5–2 mm from the ideal point of the emergence profile [11]. The correct depth positioning of a dental implant shows a 2-mm distance apical to the cement-enamel connection of the adjacent teeth (Fig. 3.1d). Periodontal surgical principles are of great importance in implantology as well as in treating natural teeth. Positioning implants

K. Kniha et al., *Guided Surgery in Implantology*, https://doi.org/10.1007/978-3-030-75216-3_3

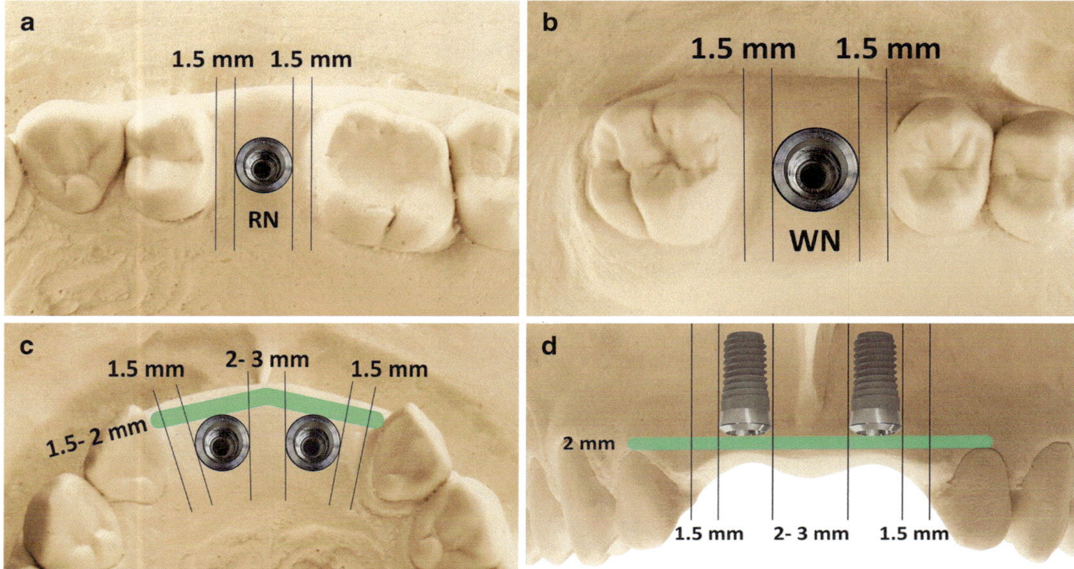

Fig. 3.1 (**a**, **b**) A distance of 1.5 mm between the implant and the neighboring teeth is obligatory (RN = regular neck). In molar positions, the use of WN (wide neck) implants can be useful. (**c**, **d**) The authors recommend a horizontal distance of 2–3 mm between two implants with a vestibular "comfort zone" of 1.5–2 mm. A 2-mm distance from the implant shoulder apical to the cement-enamel connection of the adjacent teeth represents the correct depth. (© Kristian Kniha 2021. All Rights Reserved)

too deep should be avoided, since the peri-implant pocket depth and the risk of periodontal inflammation simultaneously increase. Several studies describe the distance from the bone attachment to the adjacent tooth to the contact point of the crowns as the most important parameter, which largely influences the interdental soft tissue situation [12–19]. At a distance of ≤5 mm, a significant correlation with a full papilla could be recorded.

The exact implant position and template design will be coded in the surgical guide. Based on the implant position and axis, the sleeve diameter and sleeve position will be selected for the fabrication of the template.

Based on the virtual plan and the exactly fitting sleeve position, the surgical protocol recommends using the correct combination of drill handle cylinder and instruments for each implant (Fig. 3.2a–d). Different sleeve diameters are available, depending on the anatomical situation and the planned axis of the adjacent implants, in order to avoid sleeve collision due to inclination or narrow interdental space. Which sleeve design is used depends on the individual company. The sleeve position should be as close as possible to the gingiva and the bone while allowing for sufficient drill irrigation [20].

When successfully completed, the template design is sent to the template manufacturer. Depending on the surgeon's preference and planning system used, different surgical templates are possible: tooth-borne, gingiva-borne, or bone-borne (Table 3.1, Fig. 3.3a–d) [21].

At first, the template is attached before or during the actual implant surgery. Each template design should include inspection windows for correct position control (Fig. 3.3a). Gingiva-borne templates can optionally be placed on temporary mini-implants, and both gingiva- and bone-borne templates may be attached via small pins or screws (Fig. 3.4a, b).

The individual procedure for fabricating the scan prosthesis is dependent on the applied software and chosen template fixation (e.g., bone-, teeth- or gingiva-borne, Fig. 3.3a–d). The drilling

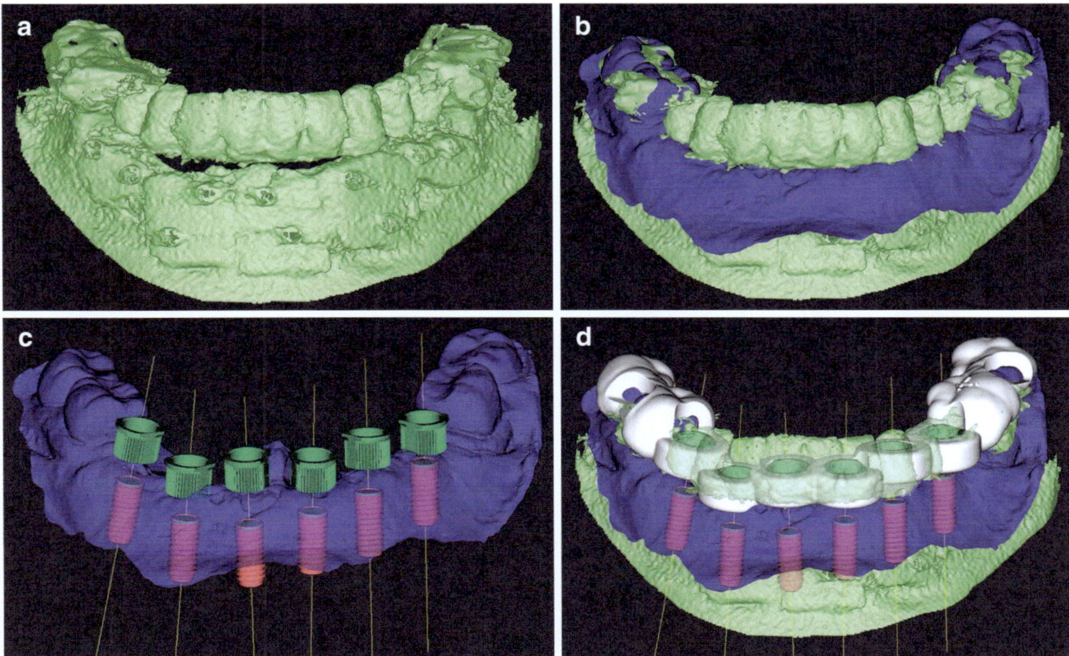

Fig. 3.2 (**a**) In this case, six dental implants in the mandible were planned using full-guided surgery. The segmented CBCT scan with the radiographic template is presented. (**b**) Matching of the 3D cast model and the CBCT scan was performed. (**c**) The implant and sleeve positions in the lower jaw were defined. (**d**) In this figure, the final planning file with the tooth-borne template for the six implants is shown. (© Kristian Kniha 2021. All Rights Reserved)

Table 3.1 Different template designs

Tooth/implant-borne templates: The surgical template is placed on the remaining teeth (existing implants).
Gingiva-borne templates: The surgical template is positioned on the mucosa. This is usually used for completely edentulous patients.
Bone-borne templates: The drilling template is placed on the bone after opening a mucous membrane flap.
Specially supported templates: The template is attached with screws or borne on temporary mini-implants. At first, the template is attached before or during the actual implant surgery.

template can additionally be stabilized with fixation pins or fixation screws or placed on temporary implants. Template production, intraoral scanning, 3D printing, radiographical inaccuracies, and template fit during surgery may lead to inaccuracies during clinical applications (Chap. 11) [21–23]. Tooth-borne templates often show the most accurate fit and support, provided that the gap width of the missing tooth or teeth is small [24].

As the gap width increases, the dental support decreases, and additional gingival support may be required. Since the mucosa has a certain resilience, inaccuracies may result from minimal descent of the template [25]. As soon as there are no teeth left, the template can be designed as either mucosa- or bone-borne. With mucosa-borne templates, the template of the upper jaw can often be positioned with sufficient accuracy due to the palatal attached mucosa [26]. In the lower jaw, on the other hand, especially if there is a lot of movable mucosa or even a flabby ridge, the exact positioning of the template may be very difficult to achieve [27]. In such cases, a bone-supported template can be considered as a third option. Optimal radiographic image quality and segmentation are essential for a proper fit of the bone-borne template [28]. A further disadvantage of bone-supported guides is the extended incision and the increased invasivity, since bone-borne

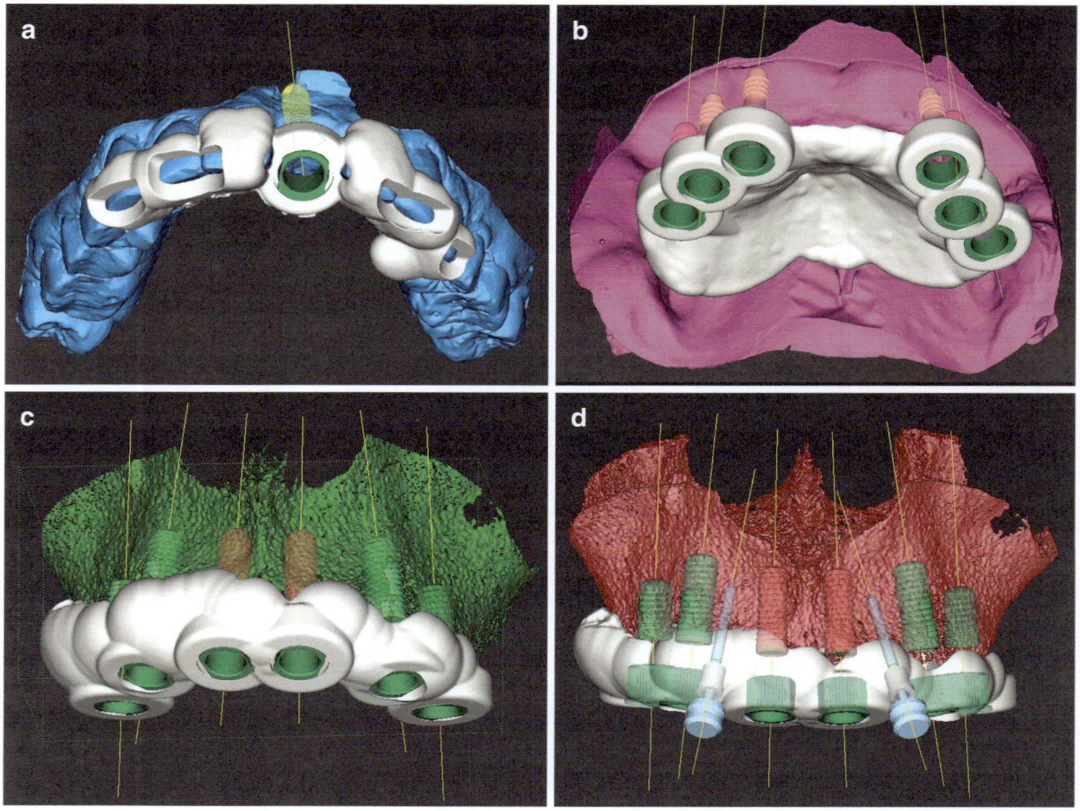

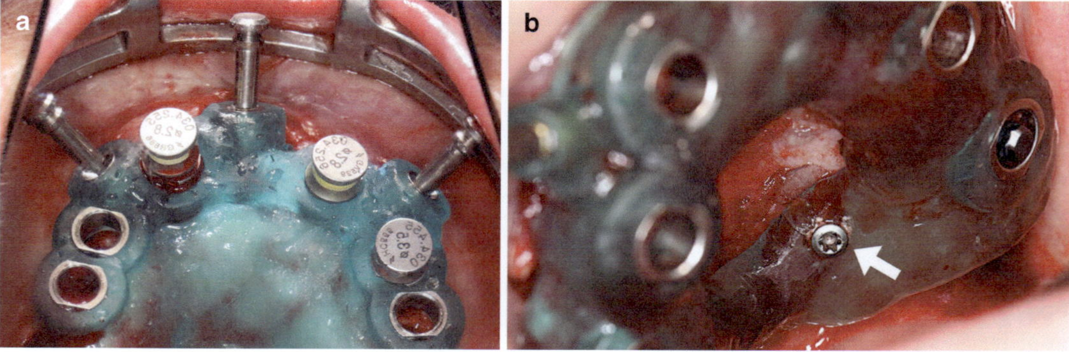

Fig. 3.3 (**a**) In the case of a tooth-borne template, the surgical guide is placed on the remaining teeth. This represents a very reliable template support. (**b**) Gingiva-borne templates are positioned on the mucosa and are usually used for completely edentulous patients. (**c**) If the drilling template is placed on the bone after opening a mucosal flap, it is called a "bone-borne template." (**d**) The guides may be secured with fixation pins or screws, as demonstrated in this planning. (© Kristian Kniha 2021, All Rights Reserved)

Fig. 3.4 (**a**) In this full-guided implant case for the upper jaw, fixation pins were used. In some systems, template fixation pins are also available; these can be inserted through the sleeves after completing the implant drilling. (**b**) In addition to pins, fixation screws may also be implemented in the guide for exact guide positioning. (© Karl Andreas Schlegel 2021. All Rights Reserved)

templates often require surgery with a larger flap for sufficient access.

The software company may act as the surgical template manufacturer, or the dental laboratory may fabricate the surgical template depending on the software concept used. The template can be produced in specialized dental laboratories or in a milling center of the program manufacturer. Depending on the manufacturer, the navigation templates are produced by stereolithography, 3D printing, or milling techniques [29]. The higher costs of 3D printing and its often limited or unproven benefits make it questionable whether it is cost-effective for all patients and applications. However, 3D medical printing has greater advantages when used to treat complex cases [30].

3.1 Conclusion

Templates may be designed as tooth-borne, gingiva-borne, or bone-borne. Tooth-borne templates show the most accurate fit and support, provided that the gap width of the missing tooth is small. When perfect implant positioning is required, especially in edentulous patients with planned fixed dentures and a lack of teeth references, full-guided surgery should be considered. However, during preoperative planning, several variables could potentially affect the accuracy of the computer-guided implant placement; one example is an intrinsic error, which can be a significant factor compared to the other factors mentioned [31].

References

1. Younes F, Cosyn J, De Bruyckere T, Cleymaet R, Bouckaert E, Eghbali A. A randomized controlled study on the accuracy of free-handed, pilot-drill guided and fully guided implant surgery in partially edentulous patients. J Clin Periodontol. 2018;45:721–32.
2. Tarnow DP, Cho SC, Wallace SS. The effect of inter-implant distance on the height of inter-implant bone crest. J Periodontol. 2000;71:546–9.
3. Teughels W, Merheb J, Quirynen M. Critical horizontal dimensions of interproximal and buccal bone around implants for optimal aesthetic out-comes: a systematic review. Clin Oral Implants Res. 2009;20(Suppl 4):134–45.
4. Degidi M, Novaes AB Jr, Nardi D, Piattelli A. Outcome analysis of immediately placed, immediately restored implants in the esthetic area: the clinical relevance of different interimplant distances. J Periodontol. 2008;79:1056–61.
5. Gastaldo JF, Cury PR, Sendyk WR. Effect of the vertical and horizontal distances between adjacent implants and between a tooth and an implant on the incidence of interproximal papilla. J Periodontol. 2004;75:1242–6.
6. De Oliveira RR, Novaes AB Jr, Papalexiou V, Muglia VA, Taba M Jr. Influence of interimplant distance on papilla formation and bone resorption: a clinical-radiographic study in dogs. J Oral Implantol. 2006;32:218–27.
7. Novaes AB Jr, Papalexiou V, Muglia V, Taba M Jr. Influence of interimplant distance on gingival papilla formation and bone resorption: clinical-radiographic study in dogs. Int J Oral Maxillofac Implants. 2006;21:45–51.
8. Kniha K, Modabber A, Kniha H, Mohlhenrich SC, Holzle F, Milz S. Dimensions of hard and soft tissue around adjacent, compared with single-tooth, zirconia implants. Br J Oral Maxillofac Surg. 2018;56:43–7.
9. Scarano A, Assenza B, Piattelli M, Thams U, San RF, Favero GA, Piattelli A. Interimplant distance and crestal bone resorption: a histologic study in the canine mandible. Clin Implant Dent Relat Res. 2004;6:150–6.
10. Kupershmidt I, Levin L, Schwartz-Arad D. Inter-implant bone height changes in anterior maxillary immediate and non-immediate adjacent dental implants. J Periodontol. 2007;78:991–6.
11. Buser D, Martin W, Belser UC. Optimizing esthetics for implant restorations in the anterior maxilla: anatomic and surgical considerations. Int J Oral Maxillofac Implants. 2004;19(Suppl):43–61.
12. Schropp L, Isidor F. Papilla dimension and soft tissue level after early vs. delayed placement of single-tooth implants: 10-year results from a randomized controlled clinical trial. Clin Oral Implants Res. 2015;26:278–86.
13. Tarnow D, Elian N, Fletcher P, Froum S, Magner A, Cho SC, Salama M, Salama H, Garber DA. Vertical distance from the crest of bone to the height of the interproximal papilla between adjacent implants. J Periodontol. 2003;74:1785–8.
14. Tarnow DP, Magner AW, Fletcher P. The effect of the distance from the contact point to the crest of bone on the presence or absence of the interproximal dental papilla. J Periodontol. 1992;63:995–56.
15. Palmer RM, Farkondeh N, Palmer PJ, Wilson RF. Astra Tech single-tooth implants: an audit of patient satisfaction and soft tissue form. J Clin Periodontol. 2007;34:633–8.
16. Kan JY, Rungcharassaeng K, Umezu K, Kois JC. Dimensions of peri-implant mucosa: an evaluation

of maxillary anterior single implants in humans. J Periodontol. 2003;74:557–62.

17. Choquet V, Hermans M, Adriaenssens P, Daelemans P, Tarnow DP, Malevez C. Clinical and radiographic evaluation of the papilla level adjacent to single-tooth dental implants. A retrospective study in the maxillary anterior region. J Periodontol. 2001;72:1364–71.

18. Kniha K, Gahlert M, Hicklin S, Bragger U, Kniha H, Milz S. Evaluation of hard and soft tissue dimensions around zirconium oxide implant-supported crowns: a 1-year retrospective study. J Periodontol. 2016;87:511–8.

19. Kniha K, Kniha H, Mohlhenrich SC, Milz S, Holzle F, Modabber A. Papilla and alveolar crest levels in immediate versus delayed single-tooth zirconia implants. Int J Oral Maxillofac Surg. 2017;46:1039–44.

20. Sannino G, Gherlone EF. Thermal changes during guided flapless implant site preparation: a comparative study. Int J Oral Maxillofac Implants. 2018;33:671–7.

21. Kuhl S, Payer M, Zitzmann NU, Lambrecht JT, Filippi A. Technical accuracy of printed surgical templates for guided implant surgery with the coDiagnostiX software. Clin Implant Dent Relat Res. 2015;17(Suppl 1):e177–82.

22. Loubele M, Van Assche N, Carpentier K, Maes F, Jacobs R, Van Steenberghe D, Suetens P. Comparative localized linear accuracy of small-field cone-beam CT and multislice CT for alveolar bone measurements. Oral Surg Oral Med Oral Pathol Oral Radiol Endod. 2008;105:512–8.

23. Behneke A, Burwinkel M, Behneke N. Factors influencing transfer accuracy of cone beam CT-derived template-based implant placement. Clin Oral Implants Res. 2012;23:416–23.

24. Pozzi A, Polizzi G, Moy PK. Guided surgery with tooth-supported templates for single missing teeth: a critical review. Eur J Oral Implantol. 2016;9(Suppl 1):S135–53.

25. Mohlhenrich SC, Brandt M, Kniha K, Prescher A, Holzle F, Modabber A, Wolf M, Peters F. Accuracy of orthodontic mini-implants placed at the anterior palate by tooth-borne or gingiva-borne guide support: a cadaveric study. Clin Oral Investig. 2019;23:4425–31.

26. Verhamme LM, Meijer GJ, Boumans T, De Haan AF, Berge SJ, Maal TJ. A clinically relevant accuracy study of computer-planned implant placement in the edentulous maxilla using mucosa-supported surgical templates. Clin Implant Dent Relat Res. 2015;17:343–52.

27. Hong J, Yun PY, Chung IH, Myoung H, Suh JD, Seo BM, Lee JH, Choung PH. Long-term follow up on recurrence of 305 ameloblastoma cases. Int J Oral Maxillofac Surg. 2007;36:283–8.

28. Marliere DAA, Demetrio MS, Picinini LS, Oliveira RG, Hdmc N. Accuracy of computer-guided surgery for dental implant placement in fully edentulous patients: a systematic review. Eur J Dent. 2018;12:153–60.

29. Vercruyssen M, Laleman I, Jacobs R, Quirynen M. Computer-supported implant planning and guided surgery: a narrative review. Clin Oral Implants Res. 2015;26(Suppl 11):69–76.

30. Tack P, Victor J, Gemmel P, Annemans L. 3D-printing techniques in a medical setting: a systematic literature review. Biomed Eng Online. 2016;15:115.

31. Cassetta M, Di Mambro A, Giansanti M, Stefanelli LV, Cavallini C. The intrinsic error of a stereolithographic surgical template in implant guided surgery. Int J Oral Maxillofac Surg. 2013;42:264–75.

Implantation with Guided Surgery (Full- vs. Half-Guided Surgery)

4

Learning Objective
- What is the process of coding the exact implant position via the guide?

If the planning is exact and the template presents an accurate fit, then an exact subsequent implant placement will usually be achieved during surgery. Each guided surgery kit is specific to the implant system. Additionally, every surgical template must be sterilizable [1]. For sterilization, follow the instructions of the template manufacturer. Damage to the material of the surgical guide should be avoided at any time. During surgery, the guide should be stored in a dry place in order to avoid material-related swelling leading to inaccuracies of fit.

Normally, the templates consist of sleeves integrated into the guide, and the individual surgical kits use handles with different heights that fit into the sleeves and individual drills that fit into the handle for implant bed preparation (Fig. 4.1a) [2]. The guided surgery kit similarly uses individual implant drills for the preparation of the implant site. The profile drill prepares the implant site for the shape of the individual implant shoulder. Thread cutting may be used according to the region and bone quality [3].

Additionally, some companies provide a stabilization system for the surgical template that uses fixation pins anchored to the template. Furthermore, instruments such as mucosa punches, milling cutters that flatten the bone (important in the case of a sharp jaw ridge),

and handpieces or ratchet adapters for full-guided implant placement are also available.

The surgical protocol, which includes the implant size and drilling sequence, is followed [4].

In this drill protocol example (Fig. 4.1b), the drill sequence for a fictitious case is shown for this particular implant system. Depending on the system, only the correct drills and handles have to be selected in relation to the individual implant position.

Implant bed preparation with guided instruments normally follows a color- or number-coded protocol, which is supplied by the manufacturer together with the surgical template or exported from the planning software. It is important to avoid the application of strong forces, especially horizontal forces, as this may lead to angular inaccuracies or easily break the guide [5]. Furthermore, the hard- and soft-tissue bedding must offer sufficient and reproducible fixation possibilities for the surgical template in the corresponding jaw [4].

Guided instruments may only be used together with the corresponding sleeves, which are fixed in templates and handles. Cutting instruments must not rotate during insertion into and removal from sleeves or handles. Ensure adequate cooling of the cutting instruments with physiologically sterile saline solution (NaCl) or Ringer's solution, using the intermittent drilling technique to avoid overheating [4]. This also applies to instruments used with handles. Information about each surgical kit of the individual manufacturer is very

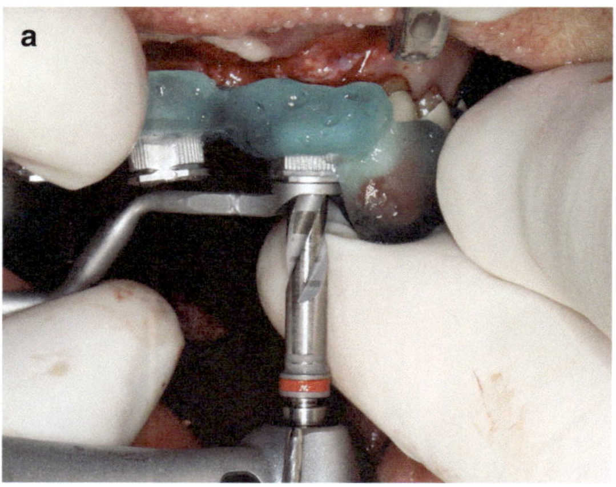

Farbkodierung	Position	Implantat-Art.-Nr.	Implantat	Hülse	Hülsenposition	Geführter Bohrer	Bohrlöffel	Planfräser
	15	021.4112 / G	SLActive Bone Level (Regular CrossFit™) Ø 4.1 mm 12 mm	H: 5 mm Ø: 5 mm	H4	≡ extra lang	••• +3 mm	3.5 mm
	13	021.4112 / G	SLActive Bone Level (Regular CrossFit™) Ø 4.1 mm 12 mm	H: 5 mm Ø: 5 mm	H4	≡ extra lang	••• +3 mm	3.5 mm
	11	021.4112 / G	SLActive Bone Level (Regular CrossFit™) Ø 4.1 mm 12 mm	H: 5 mm Ø: 5 mm	H4	≡ extra lang	••• +3 mm	3.5 mm
	21	021.4112 / G	SLActive Bone Level (Regular CrossFit™) Ø 4.1 mm 12 mm	H: 5 mm Ø: 5 mm	H4	≡ extra lang	••• +3 mm	3.5 mm
	23	021.4112 / G	SLActive Bone Level (Regular CrossFit™) Ø 4.1 mm 12 mm	H: 5 mm Ø: 5 mm	H4	≡ extra lang	••• +3 mm	3.5 mm
	25	021.4112 / G	SLActive Bone Level (Regular CrossFit™) Ø 4.1 mm 12 mm	H: 5 mm Ø: 5 mm	H4	≡ extra lang	••• +3 mm	3.5 mm

Fig. 4.1 (**a**) Application of handles with different heights that fit into the sleeves and individual drills. (**b**) Drill sequence for a fictitious case in which the extra-long drills (three dashes) and +3-mm handles (three dots) have to be selected in every implant position. In this example, the use of the drills and handles is simple; in other cases, the sequence may vary. (© Karl Andreas Schlegel 2021. All Rights Reserved)

important, as, depending on the system, pilot and twist drills may have an apical excess length (up to 0.4 mm) compared to the insertion depth of the implant.

Full-guided surgery leads to greater accuracy than with the freehand technique [6]. On the one hand, pilot drilling or complete implant bed preparation can be performed as part of half-guided surgery. With full-guided surgery, on the other hand, the implant is also inserted via the surgical guide (Fig. 4.2). According to the results of Bencharit et al. 2018 and Bover-Ramos et al. 2018, implant insertion via the template increased the accuracy [7, 8]. In addition, using guided surgery for the pilot drill was evaluated as less accurate compared to the full-guided procedure [9]. Especially when screwed dentures have been planned for implants, optimal positioning is

essential. In case of inaccuracies, it may be necessary to switch to a cemented restoration. In contrast to the studies mentioned above, there are also data that show inaccuracies in the workflow of full-guided surgery (Chap. 10) [10].

4.1 Conclusion

In full-guided surgery, from the pilot drill to implant insertion, everything is "guided." The templates consist of sleeves integrated into the guide, and the individual surgical kits use handles with different heights that fit into the sleeves and individual drills that fit into the handle for implant bed preparation. Full-guided surgery leads to greater accuracy than the half-guided or freehand techniques.

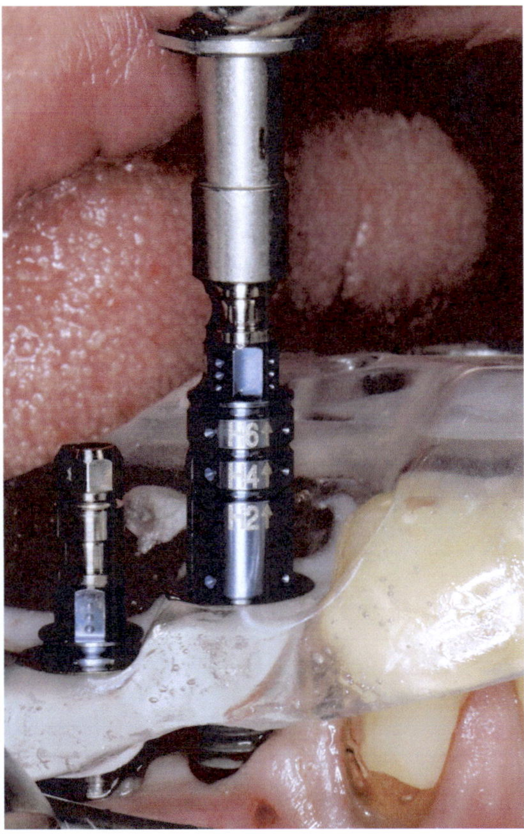

Fig. 4.2 In full-guided surgery, the implant is also inserted via the surgical guide using special insertion adapters. (© Karl Andreas Schlegel 2021. All Rights Reserved)

References

1. Ghai S, Sharma Y, Jain N, Satpathy M, Pillai AK. Use of 3-D printing technologies in craniomaxillofacial surgery: a review. Oral Maxillofac Surg. 2018;22:249–59.
2. Scherer MD, Kattadiyil MT, Parciak E, Puri S. CAD/CAM guided surgery in implant dentistry. A review of software packages and step-by-step protocols for planning surgical guides. Alpha Omegan. 2014;107:32–8.
3. Karl M, Grobecker-Karl T. Effect of bone quality, implant design, and surgical technique on primary implant stability. Quintessence Int. 2018:189–98. https://doi.org/10.3290/j.qi.a39745.
4. Al YF, Camenisch B, Al-Sabbagh M. Is digital guided implant surgery accurate and reliable? Dent Clin N Am. 2019;63:381–97.
5. Laederach V, Mukaddam K, Payer M, Filippi A, Kuhl S. Deviations of different systems for guided implant surgery. Clin Oral Implants Res. 2017;28:1147–51.
6. Tan PLB, Layton DM, Wise SL. In vitro comparison of guided versus freehand implant placement: use of a new combined TRIOS surface scanning, Implant Studio, CBCT, and stereolithographic virtually planned and guided technique. Int J Comput Dent. 2018;21:87–95.
7. Bencharit S, Staffen A, Yeung M, Whitley D 3rd, Laskin DM, Deeb GR. In vivo tooth-supported implant surgical guides fabricated with desktop stereolithographic printers: fully guided surgery is more accurate than partially guided surgery. J Oral Maxillofac Surg. 2018;76:1431–9.
8. Bover-Ramos F, Vina-Almunia J, Cervera-Ballester J, Penarrocha-Diago M, Garcia-Mira B. Accuracy of implant placement with computer-guided surgery: a systematic review and meta-analysis comparing cadaver, clinical, and in vitro studies. Int J Oral Maxillofac Implants. 2018;33:101–15.
9. Younes F, Cosyn J, De Bruyckere T, Cleymaet R, Bouckaert E, Eghbali A. A randomized controlled study on the accuracy of free-handed, pilot-drill guided and fully guided implant surgery in partially edentulous patients. J Clin Periodontol. 2018;45:721–32.
10. Flugge T, Derksen W, Te Poel J, Hassan B, Nelson K, Wismeijer D. Registration of cone beam computed tomography data and intraoral surface scans—a prerequisite for guided implant surgery with CAD/CAM drilling guides. Clin Oral Implants Res. 2017;28:1113–8.

Part II

Risk Management and Clinical Cases

Anatomical Variations and Risks During Implantation

5

Learning Objective
- Do you know the possible anatomical variations of the upper and lower jaw area?

Depending on gender, age, physique, time of edentulism, and preexisting conditions, anatomical structures vary greatly in size and bone quality [1]. The mandibula is known to have a harder structure than the maxilla because of its thicker cortical bone, whereas a greater part of the maxilla is composed of cancellous bone.

During atrophy, the resorption process of the upper arch is directed centripetally, whereas the lower jaw shrinks faster and in the centrifugal direction [2]. The progress of atrophy is partly conditioned by bone density. For clinical use, the classification of Misch et al. (D1–D4) is known to describe bone quality [3]. CBCT and CT can be useful for determining bone density at the implant recipient sites [4]. The local bone density has a predominant influence on primary implant stability, which is an important determinant factor for the individual protocol of implant loading and success [4]. Compared to implants with no peri-implant defects, a significant loss of stability should be expected when inserting implants into circular defects [5]. Furthermore, the individual thread and implant designs affect primary stability.

Inaccuracies during the guided surgery process, in particular, may lead to nerve disorders, damage anatomically important structures, and cause prosthetic complications [6]. In addition to these commonly known facts, the following passages will list severe anatomical situations that may lead to higher levels of difficulty during dental implantation.

5.1 Mandible

Due to the limitations of CBCT and CT at present, we have no option to detect nerve structures, including the trigeminal nerve. What we can usually see, on the other hand, are the boundaries of the nerve canal. Damage of the inferior alveolar nerve (N. trigeminus, N. mandibularis, and V.3), which innervates the teeth of the lower jaw and lower lip, must be avoided at any time. This nerve enters the ascending ramus of the mandible and proceeds in the mandible corpus, in its meatus. In general, within the premolar region, its withdrawal from the corpus is known as the mental nerve. In 2.2% of 3025 implant placements in the lower jaw, neurosensory damage was observed one month after implantation; however, complete recovery was observed in these patients within 13 months [7]. Furthermore, if the nerve is severely damaged (e.g., by implant drills), permanent anesthesia may result. Additionally, accessory mental foramina and loops may occur [8, 9]. CBCT imaging does improve the diagnostic protocol in patients with dental implants [7]. In a study assessing CBCT scans, the prevalence of accessory mental foramina was observed in 11.5% of the patients, and in 6.5% of all hemimandibles examined, a total of 30.0% were located anterosuperior and 23.3% posterosuperior to the mental foramen (Fig. 5.1a) [8]. Additionally, in a study published in 2017, accessory mandible canals—mostly retromolar canals—were found in 8.8% of cases [10]. In yet another study, lateral lingual foramina in the premolar area was observed in 54.3% of cases, mandibular incisive canals in 86.9%, and a loop of the inferior alveolar nerve in 14.6% of all cases (Fig. 5.1b) [9]. There are also several variants of

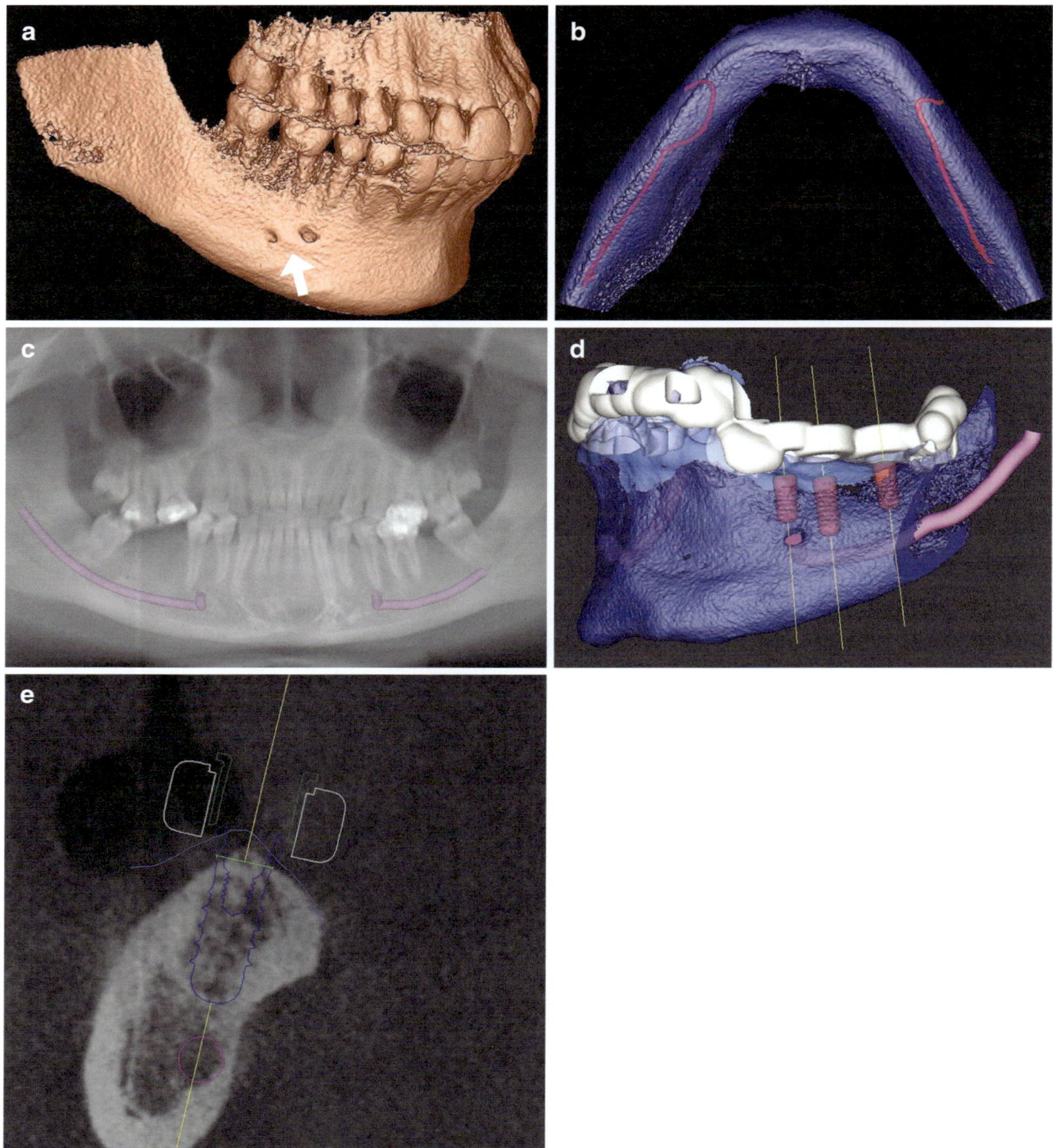

Fig. 5.1 (a) In this case, an accessory mental foramen was observed. (b) The inferior alveolar nerve may show an anterior loop before its exit through the mental foramen. (c, d) In the planning software, the inferior alveolar nerve can usually be tracked. This leads to improved visualization when positioning the implant bodies. (e) The sagittal and coronal planes should be checked for a sufficient safety distance between the bottom of the implant and the inferior alveolar nerve. (© Kristian Kniha 2021. All Rights Reserved)

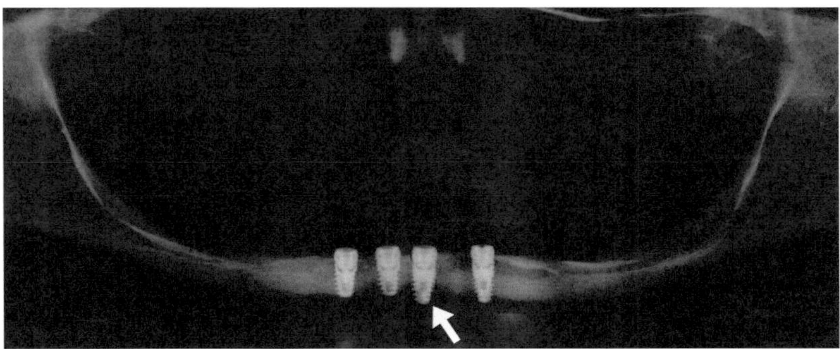

Fig. 5.2 Due to the severe atrophy of the mandible and the bicortically inserted implants (alio loco), in this case, the mandible fractured at the implant in position 32. (© Kristian Kniha 2021. All Rights Reserved)

accessory mental foramina and loops, each of which must be considered individually.

Full-guided surgery provides surgeons with enhanced diagnostic tools (visualization) for advanced implant planning (safety distance) to avoid damage of the inferior alveolar nerve (Fig. 5.1c–e).

Furthermore, a series of 151 CT scans were examined for any lingual undercuts in the posterior submandibular fossa region [11]. In 64.2% of cases, a lingual concavity was present, which can often be determined clinically by manual examination [12]. Any manifestation of a lingual undercut shape may present a risk of perforation of the lingual cortex during dental implantation. In addition to the lingual perforation with implant drills, the anterior region of the mandible depicts a risk factor for severe artery bleeding [13]. According to Balaguer-Marti et al., dental rehabilitation of the mandible canine is strongly associated with immediate and postoperative bleeding complications due to lingual cortical perforation. Cases of airway obstruction as a consequence of severe bleeding have been published [14]. In this region, the sublingual artery was found to be a branch of the lingual artery (73.5%), the submental artery (17.6%), or an anastomosis of the lingual and submental arteries (8.9%) [15]. If there is bleeding in the base of the mouth, the best way to stop it is to use a purse-string suture. The salivary ductus of the glandula sublingualis and submandibularis must not be obstructed. Optionally, a hematoma of the oral floor can also be relieved via a marginal lingual incision with drainage. If there is a risk of obstructing the airways, immedi-

ate admission to the nearest hospital is absolutely necessary to secure the airways.

Additionally, as a complication following dental implantation, spontaneous mandibular fractures are described in the literature as being associated with severely atrophied mandibles (Fig. 5.2) [16].

5.2 Maxilla

While bleeding and nerve damage are the main anatomical risk factors for implantation in the lower jaw, the main risk in the upper jaw is an injury to the adjacent paranasal sinuses. The Schneiderian membrane is the membranous lining of the maxillary sinus cavity. The maxillary sinus may be individually traversed by bony septa in the oro-vestibular direction (Fig. 5.3). Genc et al. evaluated a high prevalence of sinus septa (43.7%) in 87 CBCT maxilla scans [17]. Sinus septa have also been shown to increase the risk of incidence of Schneiderian membrane perforation during sinus lift surgery [18]. Besides a maxillary sinus lift, a nasal floor elevation may also be used for implant placement in an atrophic premaxilla [19].

5.3 Conclusion

A serious potential complication of implant surgery that can be minimized by guided implant surgery is an injury to critical anatomic structures, such as nerves, vessels, sinuses, and the nasal floor.

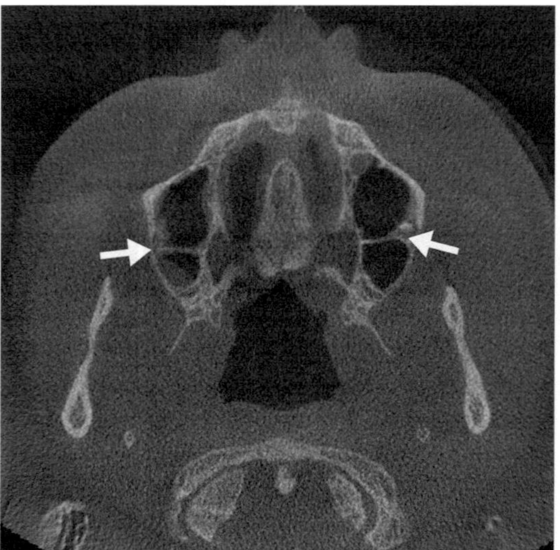

Fig. 5.3 In this CBCT scan, septa of the maxillary sinus on both sides were noticed. (© Kristian Kniha 2021. All Rights Reserved)

References

1. Di Stefano DA, Arosio P, Pagnutti S, Vinci R, Gherlone EF. Distribution of trabecular bone density in the maxilla and mandible. Implant Dent. 2019;28:340–8.
2. Klemetti E. A review of residual ridge resorption and bone density. J Prosthet Dent. 1996;75:512–4.
3. Misch CE, Dietsh-Misch F, Hoar J, Beck G, Hazen R, Misch CM. A bone quality-based implant system: first year of prosthetic loading. J Oral Implantol. 1999;25:185–97.
4. Turkyilmaz I, Mcglumphy EA. Influence of bone density on implant stability parameters and implant success: a retrospective clinical study. BMC Oral Health. 2008;8:32.
5. Ibrahim A, Heitzer M, Bock A, Peters F, Möhlhenrich SC, Hölzle F, Modabber A, Kniha K. Relationship between implant geometry and primary stability in different bony defects and variant bone densities: an in vitro study. Materials (Basel). 2020;13:4349.
6. D'haese J, Van De Velde T, Komiyama A, Hultin M, De Bruyn H. Accuracy and complications using computer-designed stereolithographic surgical guides for oral rehabilitation by means of dental implants: a review of the literature. Clin Implant Dent Relat Res. 2012;14:321–35.
7. Scarano A, Sinjari B, Murmura G, Lorusso F. Neurosensory disturbance of the inferior alveolar nerve after 3025 implant placements. Implant Dent. 2017;26:735–43.
8. Yoon TY, Ahmadi AG, Saed NA, Estrin NE, Miller DE, Dinh TN. Prevalence and anatomical characteristics of the accessory mental foramen: a study using cone beam computed tomography. Gen Dent. 2019;67:62–7.
9. Xie L, Li T, Chen J, Yin D, Wang W, Xie Z. Cone-beam CT assessment of implant-related anatomy landmarks of the anterior mandible in a Chinese population. Surg Radiol Anat. 2019;41:927–34.
10. Borgonovo AE, Taschieri S, Vavassori V, Re D, Francetti L, Corbella S. Incidence and characteristics of mandibular accessory canals: a radiographic investigation. J Investig Clin Dent. 2017;8 https://doi.org/10.1111/jicd.12260.
11. Herranz-Aparicio J, Marques J, Almendros-Marques N, Gay-Escoda C. Retrospective study of the bone morphology in the posterior mandibular region. Evaluation of the prevalence and the degree of lingual concavity and their possible complications. Med Oral Patol Oral Cir Bucal. 2016;21:e731–6.
12. Yoon TY, Patel M, Michaud RA, Manibo AM. Cone beam computerized tomography analysis of the posterior and anterior mandibular lingual concavity for dental implant patients. J Oral Implantol. 2017;43:12–8.
13. Balaguer-Marti JC, Penarrocha-Oltra D, Balaguer-Martinez J, Penarrocha-Diago M. Immediate bleeding complications in dental implants: a systematic review. Med Oral Patol Oral Cir Bucal. 2015;20:e231–8.
14. Kalpidis CD, Setayesh RM. Hemorrhaging associated with endosseous implant placement in the anterior mandible: a review of the literature. J Periodontol. 2004;75:631–45.
15. Gakonyo J, Butt F, Mwachaka P, Wagaiyu E. Arterial blood supply variation in the anterior midline mandible: significance to dental implantology. Int J Implant Dent. 2015;1:24.
16. De Groot RJ, Oomens M, Forouzanfar T, Schulten E. Bone augmentation followed by implant surgery in the edentulous mandible: a systematic review. J Oral Rehabil. 2018;45:334–43.
17. Genc T, Duruel O, Kutlu HB, Dursun E, Karabulut E, Tozum TF. Evaluation of anatomical structures and variations in the maxilla and the mandible before dental implant treatment. Dent Med Probl. 2018;55:233–40.
18. Al-Dajani M. Incidence, risk factors, and complications of schneiderian membrane perforation in sinus lift surgery: a meta-analysis. Implant Dent. 2016;25:409–15.
19. Garcia-Denche JT, Abbushi A, Hernandez G, Fernandez-Tresguerres I, Lopez-Cabarcos E, Tamimi F. Nasal floor elevation for implant treatment in the atrophic premaxilla: a within-patient comparative study. Clin Implant Dent Relat Res. 2015;17(Suppl 2):e520–30.

6

Complications, Inaccuracies, and Sources of Error in Full-Guided Surgery

Learning Objective
- What can go wrong when using guided surgery?

Full-guided surgery includes the process of digital planning, fabrication of the individual template, and implant placement using the surgical template and a specific guided surgery kit. However, there are numerous additional steps that go beyond the initial prosthetic diagnosis, treatment planning, and surgical template fabrication. Significant errors can occur and accumulate during each of these individual steps, which may significantly affect the final accuracy and produce enormous deviations from correct implant placement [1].

6.1 CBCT and CT Imaging, Impression, and Oral Scan

A variation in diagnostic image quality, showing a substantial variability between CBCT technologies and exposure protocols, has been described in the literature [2]. A resolution of 0.2 voxels has been ascribed to CBCT imaging [2]. Furthermore, the measurement error within CBCT scans was assessed to be up to 0.26 mm for linear distances [3]. From the point of view of accuracy, a protocol with high spatial resolution is absolutely necessary to achieve the best radiographic results. However, the factor that has the greatest influence on accuracy is the segmentation of the CBCT data and not the scan itself [4]. It means that the more precise the segmentation, the higher the achieved accuracy will be.

According to Schnutenhaus et al., the accuracy of the extraoral scanner used on the cast models is specified by the manufacturer as less than 20 µm [2]. As the extension increases to cover the entire quadrant, the inferiority of the optical impressions becomes more apparent [5, 6]. Additionally, the mean impression inaccuracy of A-silicone was measured up to 62 µm and can therefore be ignored, as the resolution of the CBCT is 0.2 voxels [7].

Intraoral scanners from different companies showed different standard deviations and thus different accuracies during the digital impression [5, 6]. The inaccuracies of all oral scan systems increase with the extension of the area to be captured, from single-tooth gaps to entire jaw sections. When scanning one jaw, a deviation tolerance of 17–378 µm is to be expected.

6.2 Planning Software

The manual segmentation of 3D models by the user proved to be significantly better than automatic segmentation, especially for patients with metallic restorations [8]. Between the virtual teeth model and the CBCT model, an overall deviation of 0.54 mm was found in one study [8]. According to the results of Ritter et al. from 2012, data matching of a 3D surface and CBCT scans works reliably and is sufficiently accurate

© The Author(s), under exclusive license to Springer Nature Switzerland AG 2021
K. Kniha et al., *Guided Surgery in Implantology*, https://doi.org/10.1007/978-3-030-75216-3_6

for dental implant planning, with inaccuracies up to 0.14 mm (SD = 0.18 mm) [9]. In cases where many artifacts are expected due to an excess of metallic restorations, the use of an X-ray template may still be indicated [2]. Superposition errors are low when CBCT and optical scans of buccal and lingual tooth surfaces are used for matching [10]. Additionally, the authors suggest that the dentition of the upper and lower jaw should be separated in every CBCT scan.

In contrast to the matching operation, it is unlikely that the template fabrication process has a significant impact on the overall accuracy of a stereolithographic template [4]. The accuracy of 3D printers today is stated to be less than 200 µm, which corresponds to the resolution of CBCT scans [11].

6.3 Surgical Template

Tooth-borne templates constitute a favorable guide design regarding accuracy. On the other hand, gingiva-borne surgical guides used in the treatment of completely edentulous maxillae showed that angular and linear deviations are to be expected [4]. This agrees with the results of Möhlenrich et al. who calculated statistical differences in lateral deviations between tooth- and gingiva-borne templates of 0.88 and 1.65 mm, respectively. Between both template designs no differences were found in the vertical deviations, however, both the tooth- and gingiva-borne templates exhibited high inaccuracies of 2.34 and 2.14 mm, respectively [12]. In contrast to virtual planning, postoperative oral scans and CBCT scans reflected diverging measures of accuracy [13]. A systematic review concluded that bone-borne surgical guides have the highest inaccuracy compared to other types of guides [14].

6.4 Guided Surgery

Movements or the incorrect positioning of the drilling template during implant preparation could lead to inaccuracy [15]. However, this is more likely to be the case with mucosa-supported drilling templates [16]. Therefore, guides supported by mini-implants during surgery have demonstrated high accuracy in implant positioning [14]. Another study has also shown that drills and sleeves have a certain freedom of movement and are therefore slightly prone to lateral deviations of the implants [17]. It is essential to avoid the use of excessive force during surgery.

6.5 Overall Accuracy

During full-guided surgery, for the entire manufacturing process, deviations of up to 0.7 mm may occur [4]. This value agrees with another study, which found a maximum inaccuracy of 0.72 mm between the planned and actual implant positions in the apical direction [18]. Derksen et al. also suggested that a vertical safety margin to important anatomic structures, such as the inferior alveolar nerve, of 1.5 mm is necessary. In the 2014 study of Vercruyssen et al., the inaccuracy of template-guided surgery (with a mean deviation at the entry point of 1.4 mm and an angular deviation of 3.0°) was significantly less than in non-template-guided surgery (2.8 mm and an angular deviation of 9.1°) [19]. From these findings, Vercruyssen et al. concluded that guided surgery has an added value, but at each step, awareness of possible deviation errors is crucial for the success of treatment. However, there are contradictory statements in the current literature. According to Pozzi et al., no statistically significant differences were observed between guided surgery and freehand implantation, except for more postoperative pain and swelling in freehand-treated areas, as the flaps were more often elevated (Table 6.1) [20].

6.6 Conclusion

Guided surgery is a practical treatment option for which the literature shows support in terms of accuracy. However, deviations do occur and have a significant impact on the final implant accuracy.

Table 6.1 Overview of risks that may affect accuracy during guided surgery

Workflow guided surgery	Inaccuracies and complications	Prevention
CBCT and CT imaging	• Image quality (artifacts) • Template fit inaccuracy • Patient's movement during the scan • Contact of teeth during the scan	• If possible, avoid metal structures in the field of view • Patient instruction • Bite on cotton wool rolls
Planning software	• Incorrect digital implant placement • Inaccurate software matching	• Correct implant position (Chap. 3) • Clear matching references
Surgical template	• Incorrect guide position or movement • Different guide designs	• Appropriate fixation and fit check • Attention with gingiva- and bone-borne templates
Guided surgery	• Insufficient mouth opening • Guide fracture or drill overuse • Overheating	• Important in the posterior area • Avoid high forces • Sufficient irrigation

References

1. Tatakis DN, Chien HH, Parashis AO. Guided implant surgery risks and their prevention. Periodontology. 2019;2000(81):194–208.
2. Schnutenhaus S, Groller S, Luthardt RG, Rudolph H. Accuracy of the match between cone beam computed tomography and model scan data in template-guided implant planning: a prospective controlled clinical study. Clin Implant Dent Relat Res. 2018;20:541–9.
3. Mischkowski RA, Pulsfort R, Ritter L, Neugebauer J, Brochhagen HG, Keeve E, Zoller JE. Geometric accuracy of a newly developed cone-beam device for maxillofacial imaging. Oral Surg Oral Med Oral Pathol Oral Radiol Endod. 2007;104:551–9.
4. D'haese J, Van De Velde T, Komiyama A, Hultin M, De Bruyn H. Accuracy and complications using computer-designed stereolithographic surgical guides for oral rehabilitation by means of dental implants: a review of the literature. Clin Implant Dent Relat Res. 2012;14:321–35.
5. Rutkunas V, Geciauskaite A, Jegelevicius D, Vaitiekunas M. Accuracy of digital implant impressions with intraoral scanners. A systematic review. Eur J Oral Implantol. 2017;10(Suppl 1):101–20.
6. Abduo J, Elseyoufi M. Accuracy of intraoral scanners: a systematic review of influencing factors. Eur J Prosthodont Restor Dent. 2018;26:101–21.
7. Rudolph H, Quaas S, Haim M, Preissler J, Walter MH, Koch R, Luthardt RG. Randomized controlled clinical trial on the three-dimensional accuracy of fast-set impression materials. Clin Oral Investig. 2013;17:1397–406.
8. Flugge T, Derksen W, Te Poel J, Hassan B, Nelson K, Wismeijer D. Registration of cone beam computed tomography data and intraoral surface scans—a prerequisite for guided implant surgery with CAD/CAM drilling guides. Clin Oral Implants Res. 2017;28:1113–8.
9. Ritter L, Reiz SD, Rothamel D, Dreiseidler T, Karapetian V, Scheer M, Zoller JE. Registration accuracy of three-dimensional surface and cone beam computed tomography data for virtual implant planning. Clin Oral Implants Res. 2012;23:447–52.
10. Noh H, Nabha W, Cho JH, Hwang HS. Registration accuracy in the integration of laser-scanned dental images into maxillofacial cone-beam computed tomography images. Am J Orthod Dentofac Orthop. 2011;140:585–91.
11. Neumeister A, Schulz L, Glodecki C. Investigations on the accuracy of 3D-printed drill guides for dental implantology. Int J Comput Dent. 2017;20:35–51.
12. Mohlhenrich SC, Brandt M, Kniha K, Prescher A, Holzle F, Modabber A, Wolf M, Peters F. Accuracy of orthodontic mini-implants placed at the anterior palate by tooth-borne or gingiva-borne guide support: a cadaveric study. Clin Oral Investig. 2019;23:4425–31.
13. Kniha K, Brandt M, Bock A, Modabber A, Prescher A, Hölzle F, Danesh G, Möhlhenrich SC. Accuracy of fully guided orthodontic mini-implant placement evaluated by cone-beam computed tomography: a study involving human cadaver heads. Clin Oral Investig. 2021;25:1299–306.
14. Tahmaseb A, Wismeijer D, Coucke W, Derksen W. Computer technology applications in surgical implant dentistry: a systematic review. Int J Oral Maxillofac Implants. 2014;29(Suppl):25–42.
15. Di Giacomo GA, Cury PR, De Araujo NS, Sendyk WR, Sendyk CL. Clinical application of stereolithographic surgical guides for implant placement: preliminary results. J Periodontol. 2005;76:503–7.
16. Cassetta M, Di Mambro A, Giansanti M, Stefanelli LV, Cavallini C. The intrinsic error of a stereolithographic surgical template in implant guided surgery. Int J Oral Maxillofac Surg. 2013;42:264–75.
17. Koop R, Vercruyssen M, Vermeulen K, Quirynen M. Tolerance within the sleeve inserts of different surgical guides for guided implant surgery. Clin Oral Implants Res. 2013;24:630–4.

18. Derksen W, Wismeijer D, Flugge T, Hassan B, Tahmaseb A. The accuracy of computer-guided implant surgery with tooth-supported, digitally designed drill guides based on CBCT and intra-oral scanning. A prospective cohort study. Clin Oral Implants Res. 2019;30:1005–15.
19. Vercruyssen M, Cox C, Coucke W, Naert I, Jacobs R, Quirynen M. A randomized clinical trial comparing guided implant surgery (bone- or mucosa-supported) with mental navigation or the use of a pilot-drill template. J Clin Periodontol. 2014;41:717–23.
20. Pozzi A, Polizzi G, Moy PK. Guided surgery with tooth-supported templates for single missing teeth: a critical review. Eur J Oral Implantol. 2016;9 (Suppl 1):S135–53.

Learning Objective
- What should be considered in full-arch cases with removable versus fixed dentures?

Especially in patients with complete tooth loss and a lack of surgical reference points, full-guided surgery may be of enormous importance and help for ideal implant placement. The current literature supports the use of multiple implant numbers for either fixed- or removable-tooth restorations in full-arch cases [1]. It means there exists a recommended range regarding the implant number for either fixed or removable dentures.

Nevertheless, the Consensus Conference on Implantology of various German associations (e.g., the Bundesverband der implantologisch tätigen Zahnärzte in Europa e.V., Deutsche Gesellschaft für Implantologie im Zahn-, Mund- und Kieferbereich e.V., Deutsche Gesellschaft für zahnärztliche Implantologie e.V., Deutsche Gesellschaft für Mund-, Kiefer- und Gesichtschirurgie e.V. und Berufsverband der Oralchirurgen e.V.) has described indication classes in implantology in relation to the initial situation and the development of the field in the meantime [2]. It states that "the optimal therapy of replacing every tooth with an implant cannot always be carried out for various reasons (especially anatomical, but also economic reasons). Additionally, the necessity of the replacement of the seventh tooth has to be critically assessed individually. Deviations from this standard in the number of implants are not inevitably wrong. There are many reasons why a patient does not want to opt for a higher quality implant-supported restoration or, conversely, why an increase in the number of implants compared to the standard number is medically necessary.

There are different forms of restoration as treatment compromises in individual cases with implant numbers other than those noted below for the standard case, particularly in order to avoid surgical interventions that increase the existing jaw bone supply (e.g., short implants, angulated implants, implants with reduced diameter)" [2].

The indication class of edentulous patients suggested using six implants for removable and eight implants for fixed prostheses in the upper jaw. On the other hand, four implants for removable and six implants for fixed prostheses should be used in the lower jaw.

Many factors have been shown to influence the individual implant count for either removable or fixed dentures; however, the authors feel that the recommendation for implant numbers in fixed and removable dentures shows a good compromise between a minimum number and an oversupply of implants.

Patients often wish to receive an implant-supported fixed prosthesis in edentulous cases [3]. However, fixed prosthetic rehabilitation, especially of the edentulous maxilla, is known to be challenging and requires careful planning. Therefore, a temporary tooth setup without the anterior labial flange, in which the esthetics can be assessed, should be fabricated first [4]. Based on this initial analysis, an individual decision should be made whether to use a crown- or bridge-based fixed prosthesis or a removable hybrid prosthesis with the use of gingiva-colored material [4].

The prosthetic designs in full-arch cases differ mainly in the type of retention, the prosthetic material mix, the framework design, and the use of gingiva-colored denture material.

Previous authors have addressed issues related to treatment planning of the edentulous upper jaw for fixed dentures, such as esthetic challenges, including the lip support and smile line (Fig. 7.1a, b) [5, 6]. Zitzmann et al. suggested the alternative use of a removable denture, such as an overdenture supported by a bar or individual attachments [5, 6]. With a sufficient number of implants, a removable denture may be designed almost "fixed," and this type of denture can be removed by the patient for hygienic reasons. More importantly, the need for gingiva material in fixed dentures may produce plaque accumulating areas, which may lead to peri-implantitis.

However, in special cases, a crown- or bridge-based denture is realizable. Block et al. showed that for a crown- or bridge-based prosthesis without any gingiva material, the vertical position of the edentulous ridge should be on the level of the smile line, and the planned teeth have to be directly on the alveolar ridge [7]. In case of a wrong smile line or insufficient support, surgeons should switch to a removable hybrid denture. The case in Fig. 7.1 is an example where a removable prosthesis has been chosen, as the upper part presented insufficient support according to the criteria of Black et al. Furthermore, using the anterior labial flange, the smile line was set correctly.

In cases in which the smile line is located near the alveolar ridge (Fig. 7.2a–c), a crown- or bridge-based fixed prosthesis may be chosen. In this patient, lip support was sufficient and a fixed prosthesis could be realized. If the alveolar ridge is located more incisively when compared to the smile line, an osteotomy might be indicated to improve the excessive gingival display, also called a "gummy smile."

7.1   Conclusion

One may choose a crown- or bridge-based prosthesis without any gingiva material in the maxilla, with the vertical position of the edentulous ridge at the level of the smile line and with the planned teeth directly on the alveolar ridge. Otherwise, a removable hybrid prosthesis should be recommended.

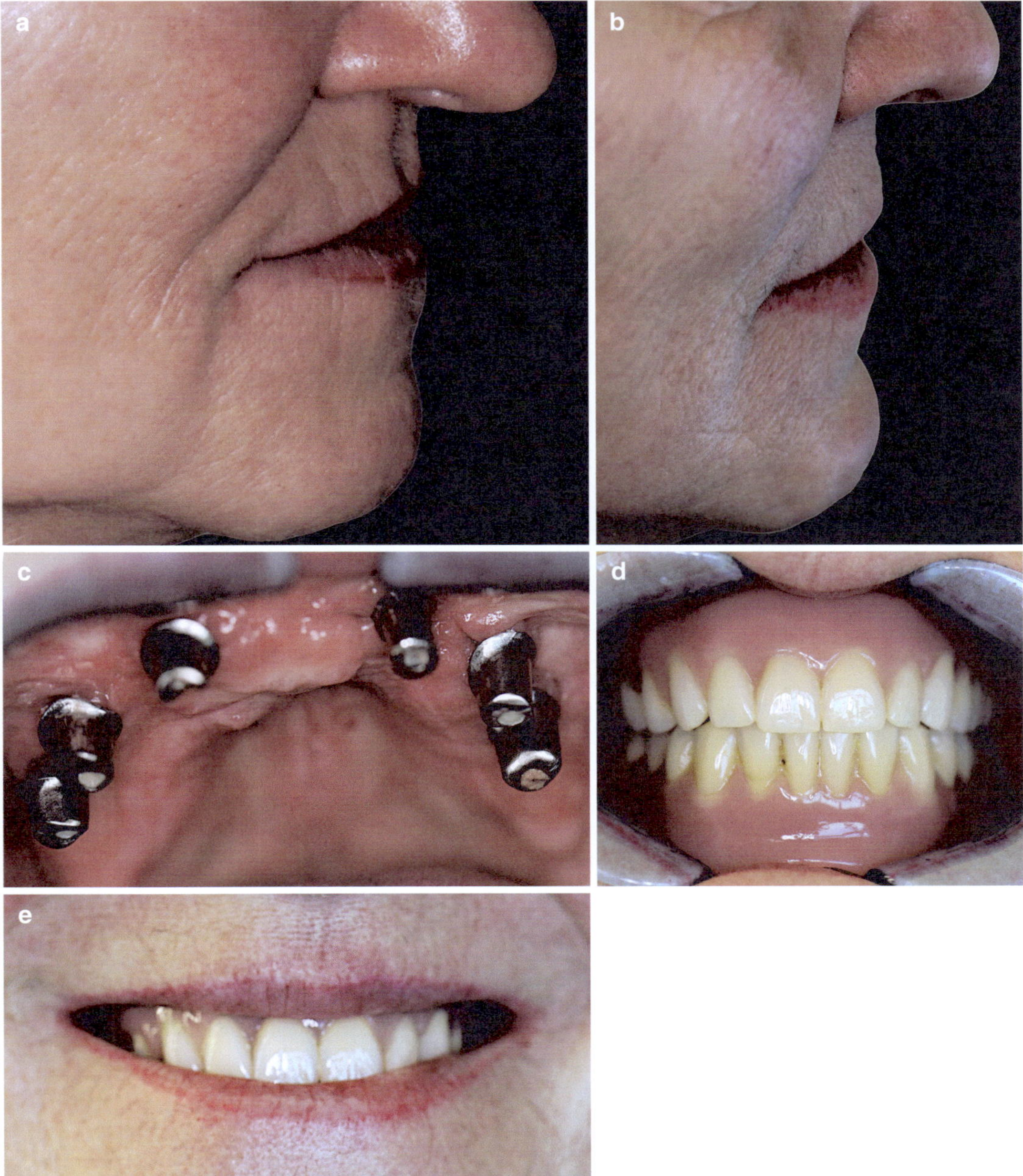

Fig. 7.1 (**a**) In this case, the patient presented a negative lip profile without any teeth. (**b**) After insertion of the final removable prosthesis, the lip profile was corrected. (**c**) The anterior labial flange of the denture was used to improve the lip profile. For optimal oral hygiene, such dentures should be fabricated as removable prostheses. (**d**) Using six implants with telescopic attachments in the maxilla, the hybrid prostheses showed a very high retention. (**e**) Using the anterior labial flange, a correct smile line was created. (© Karl Andreas Schlegel 2021. All Rights Reserved)

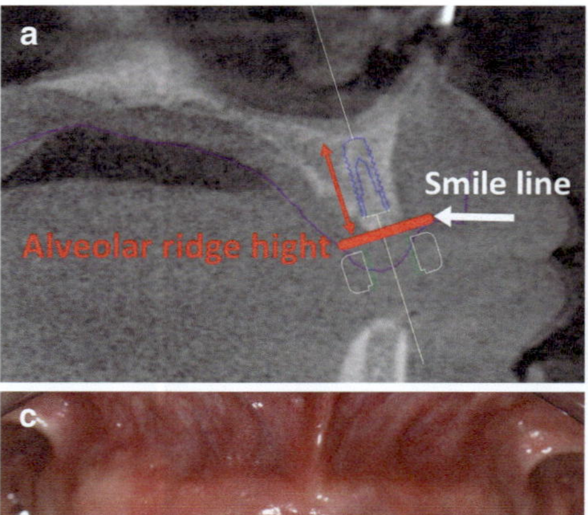

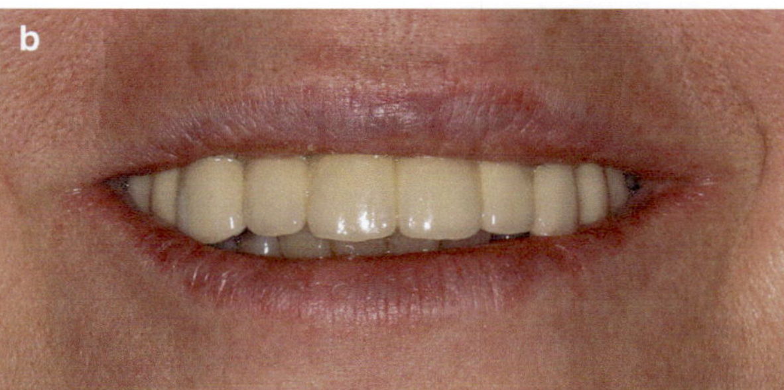

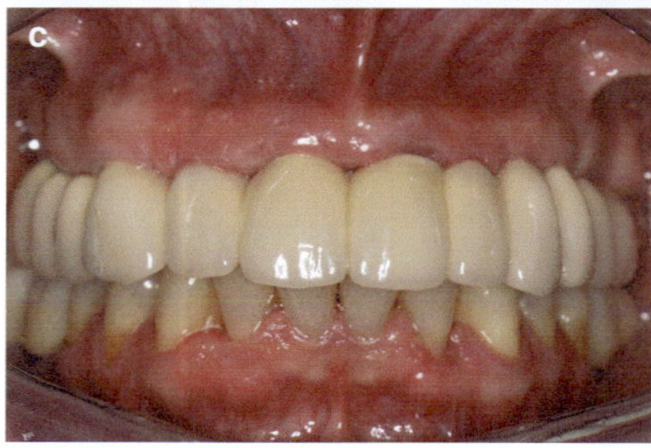

Fig. 7.2 (**a**) When considering a crown- or bridge-based fixed prosthesis, the smile line should at least present the level of the alveolar ridge, and the exact planned tooth position should be located directly on the alveolar ridge. (**b**, **c**) Due to the individual smile line near the alveolar ridge height, a crown- or bridge-based fixed prosthesis could be performed in this case. (© Karl Andreas Schlegel 2021. All Rights Reserved)

References

1. Morton D, Gallucci G, Lin WS, Pjetursson B, Polido W, Roehling S, Sailer I, Aghaloo T, Albera H, Bohner L, Braut V, Buser D, Chen S, Dawson A, Eckert S, Gahlert M, Hamilton A, Jaffin R, Jarry C, Karayazgan B, Laine J, Martin W, Rahman L, Schlegel A, Shiota M, Stilwell C, Vorster C, Zembic A, Zhou W. Group 2 ITI consensus report: prosthodontics and implant dentistry. Clin Oral Implants Res. 2018;29(Suppl 16):215–23.

2. Bundesverband Der Implantologisch Tätigen Zahnärzte in Europa e.V. (Bdiz Edi), Deutsche Gesellschaft Für Implantologie Im Zahn- Mund- Und Kieferbereich e.V. (Dgi), Deutsche Gesellschaft Für Zahnärztliche Implantologie e.V. (Dgzi), Deutsche Gesellschaft Für Mund- Kiefer- Und Gesichtschirurgie e.V. (Dgmkg), Berufsverband Der Oralchirurgen e.V. (Bdo). Konsensuskonferenz Implantologie—Indikationsbeschreibung für die Regelfallversorgung in der Implantologie. 2014. https://www.konsensuskonferenz-implantologie.eu/wp-content/uploads/141125_Indikationsklassen.pdf

3. Bedrossian E, Sullivan RM, Fortin Y, Malo P, Indresano T. Fixed-prosthetic implant restoration of the edentulous maxilla: a systematic pretreatment evaluation method. J Oral Maxillofac Surg. 2008;66:112–22.

4. Bidra AS. Three-dimensional esthetic analysis in treatment planning for implant-supported fixed prosthesis in the edentulous maxilla: review of the esthetics literature. J Esthet Restor Dent. 2011;23:219–36.

5. Zitzmann NU, Marinello CP. Treatment plan for restoring the edentulous maxilla with implant-supported restorations: removable overdenture versus fixed partial denture design. J Prosthet Dent. 1999;82:188–96.

6. Zitzmann NU, Marinello CP. Treatment outcomes of fixed or removable implant-supported prostheses in the edentulous maxilla. Part II: clinical findings. J Prosthet Dent. 2000;83:434–42.

7. Block MS. Maxillary fixed prosthesis design based on the preoperative physical examination. J Oral Maxillofac Surg. 2015;73:851–60.

Guided Surgery with Tooth-Supported Templates: Clinical Cases

Guided implantology surely has several advantages. Full-guided surgery in dental implantology will further improve over the next decade and is going to provide surgeons with enhanced diagnostic tools for advanced implant planning. The current protocol of guided surgery enables prosthetically oriented implant backward planning and subsequent implant placement. Full-guided surgery usually consists of the following steps: clinical preparation and medical imaging, data collection and software planning, fabrication of the guide, full-guided implantation, and, in selected cases, immediate prosthodontic restoration.

Although it may be assumed that guided implantology is always 100% precise and reliable compared to free implant placement, due to the surgical learning curve and possible accumulated errors that may occur during the various steps of the process, there may be inaccuracies. Therefore, a definitive immediate treatment is not recommended in the current literature. The use of guided surgery should not lead to a template-based implant placement without any control. Based on the available literature, there is no clear evidence that computer-guided surgery is superior to conventional procedures. Of course, new developments will have a further positive impact on guided surgery. More randomized clinical long-term data regarding guided implantology are necessary.

In the next chapters, we would like to discuss various initial situations and treatment options on the subject of guided surgery. For this purpose, we will present a number of clinical cases.

K. Kniha et al., *Guided Surgery in Implantology*, https://doi.org/10.1007/978-3-030-75216-3_8

8.1   Case I: Flapless (Figs. 8.1, 8.2, 8.3, 8.4, 8.5, 8.6, and 8.7)

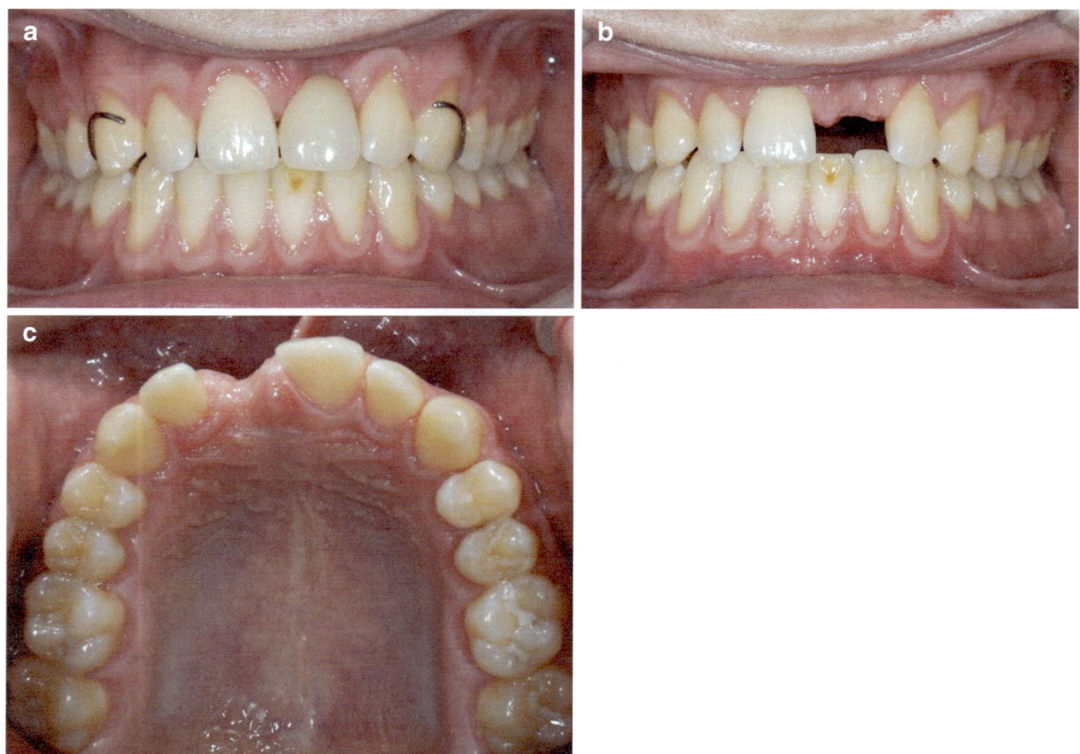

Fig. 8.1 (**a–c**) In this example, a hard tissue deficit characterized the initial situation, in which tooth loss occurred in region 21. (© Karl Andreas Schlegel 2021. All Rights Reserved)

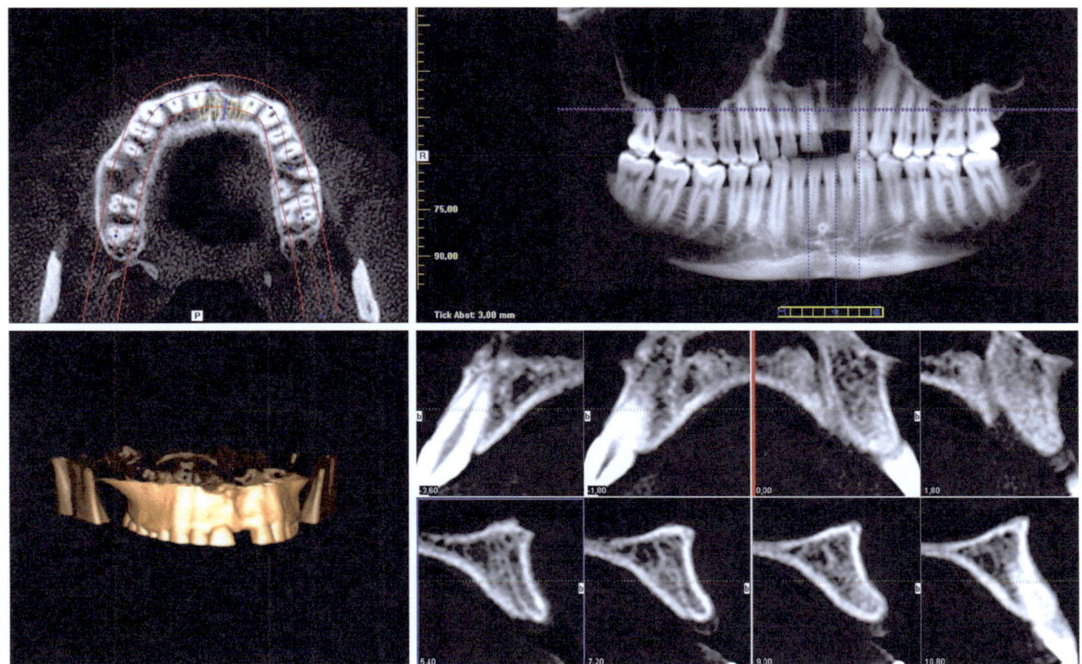

Fig. 8.2 The three-dimensional X-ray examination showed an insufficient bone bed, which first had to be augmented before implantation. (© Karl Andreas Schlegel 2021. All Rights Reserved)

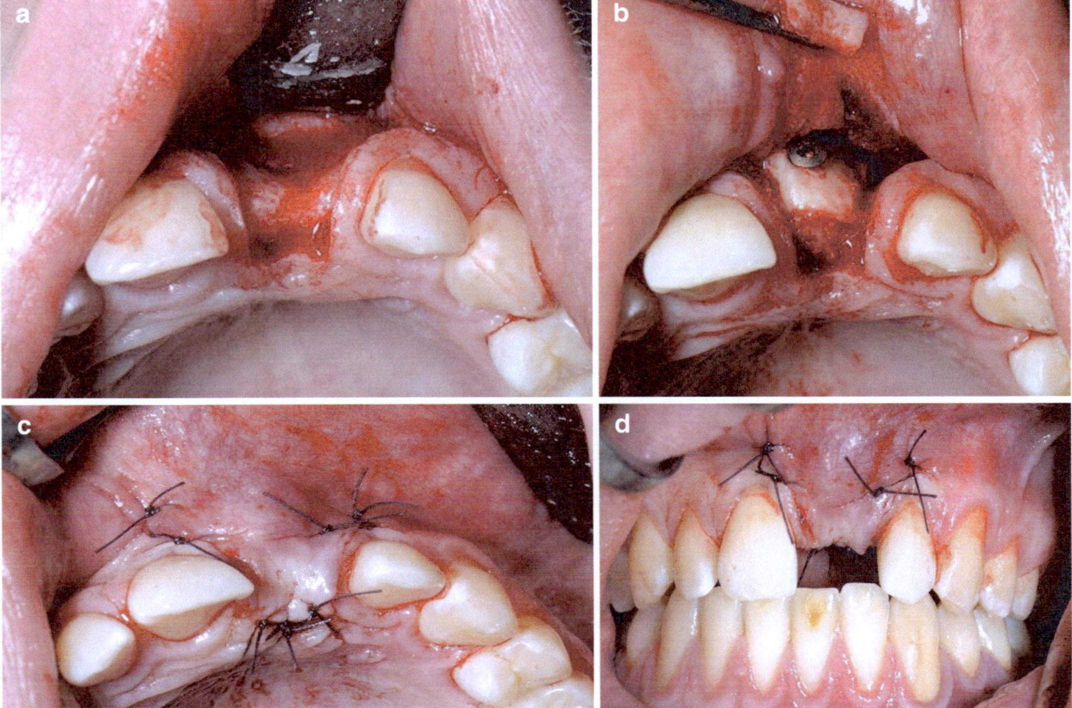

Fig. 8.3 (**a–d**) Here, an autologous cortical bone harvest from the retromolar region of the lower jaw was chosen. The bone block was fixed using an osteosynthesis screw. (© Karl Andreas Schlegel 2021. All Rights Reserved)

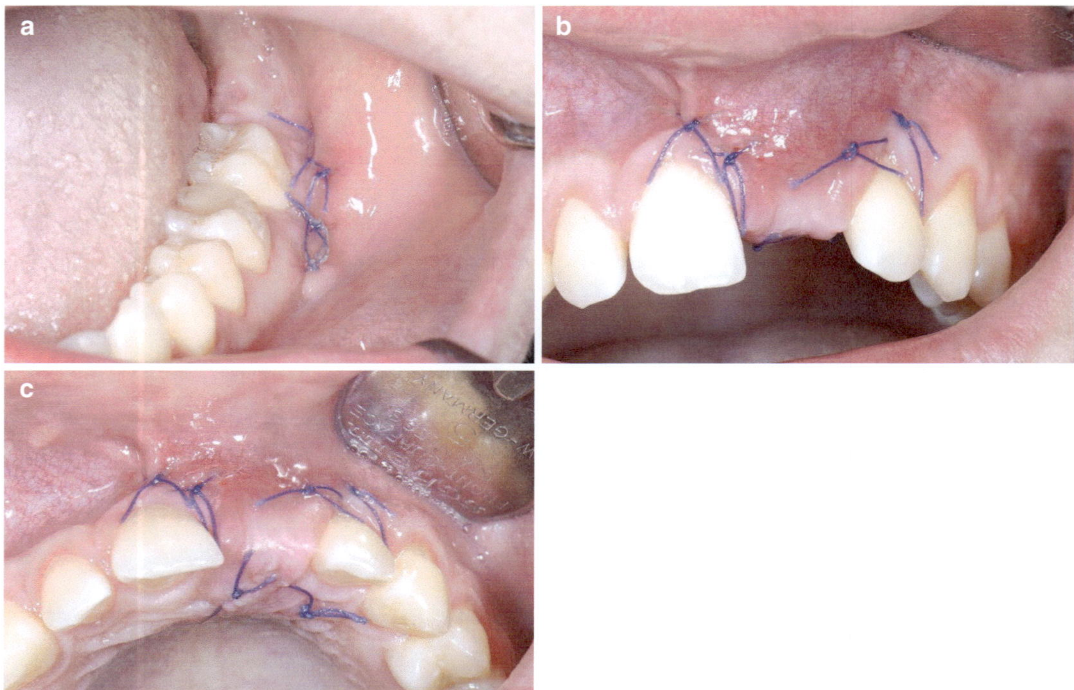

Fig. 8.4 (a–c) After 7 days, the wound presented signs of regular healing. (© Karl Andreas Schlegel 2021. All Rights Reserved)

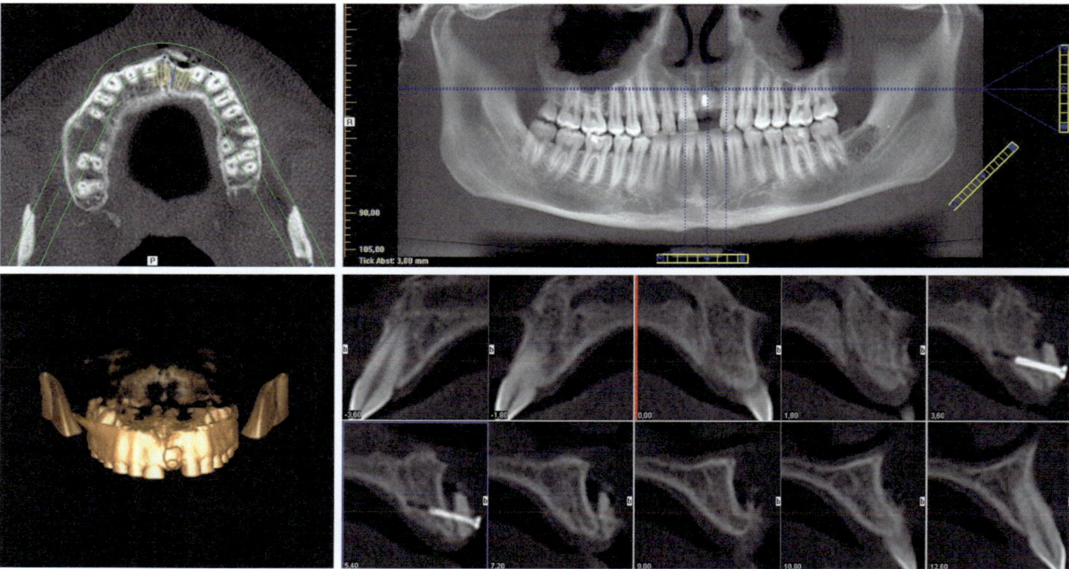

Fig. 8.5 The successful osseous augmentation now revealed sufficient volume for guided implant placement. (© Karl Andreas Schlegel 2021. All Rights Reserved)

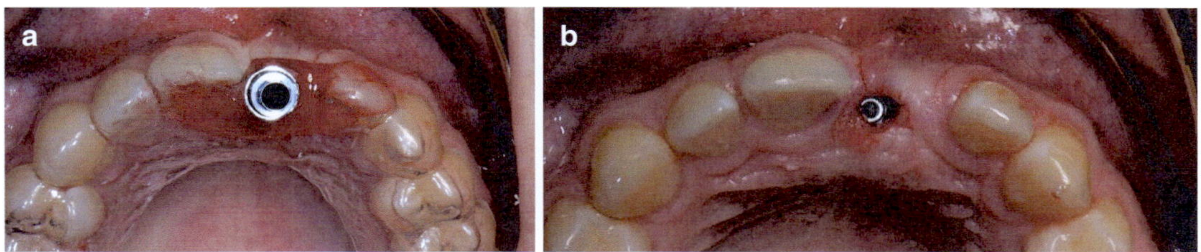

Fig. 8.6 (**a**, **b**) After checking the fit of the splint, the implant could be inserted with a tooth-borne template. (© Karl Andreas Schlegel 2021. All Rights Reserved)

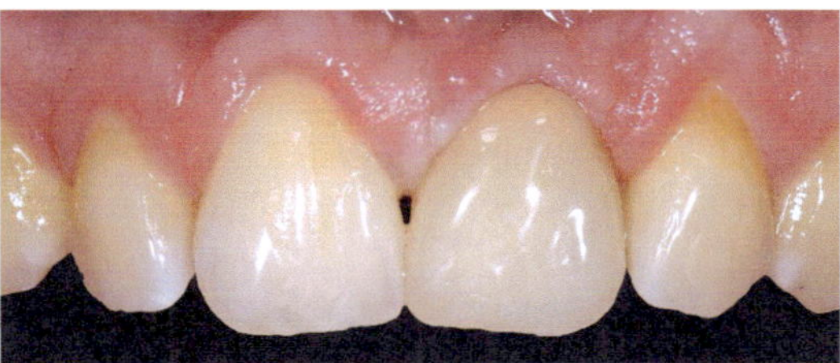

Fig. 8.7 Final result after 1 year of follow-up. (© Karl Andreas Schlegel 2021. All Rights Reserved)

8.2   Case II: Flapless (Figs. 8.8, 8.9, 8.10, 8.11, and 8.12)

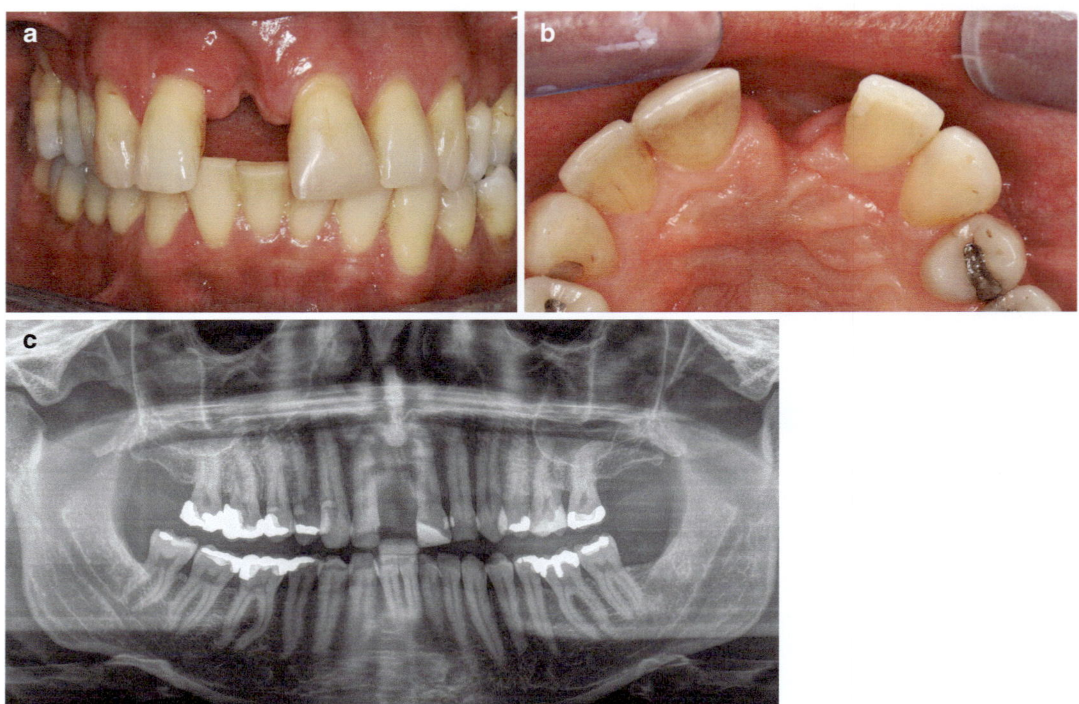

Fig. 8.8 (a–c) A hard tissue deficit characterizes the initial situation in this case example, in which, again, tooth loss occurred in region 21. Additionally, the risk of gingival recession in this young man aggravates the case. (© Karl Andreas Schlegel 2021. All Rights Reserved)

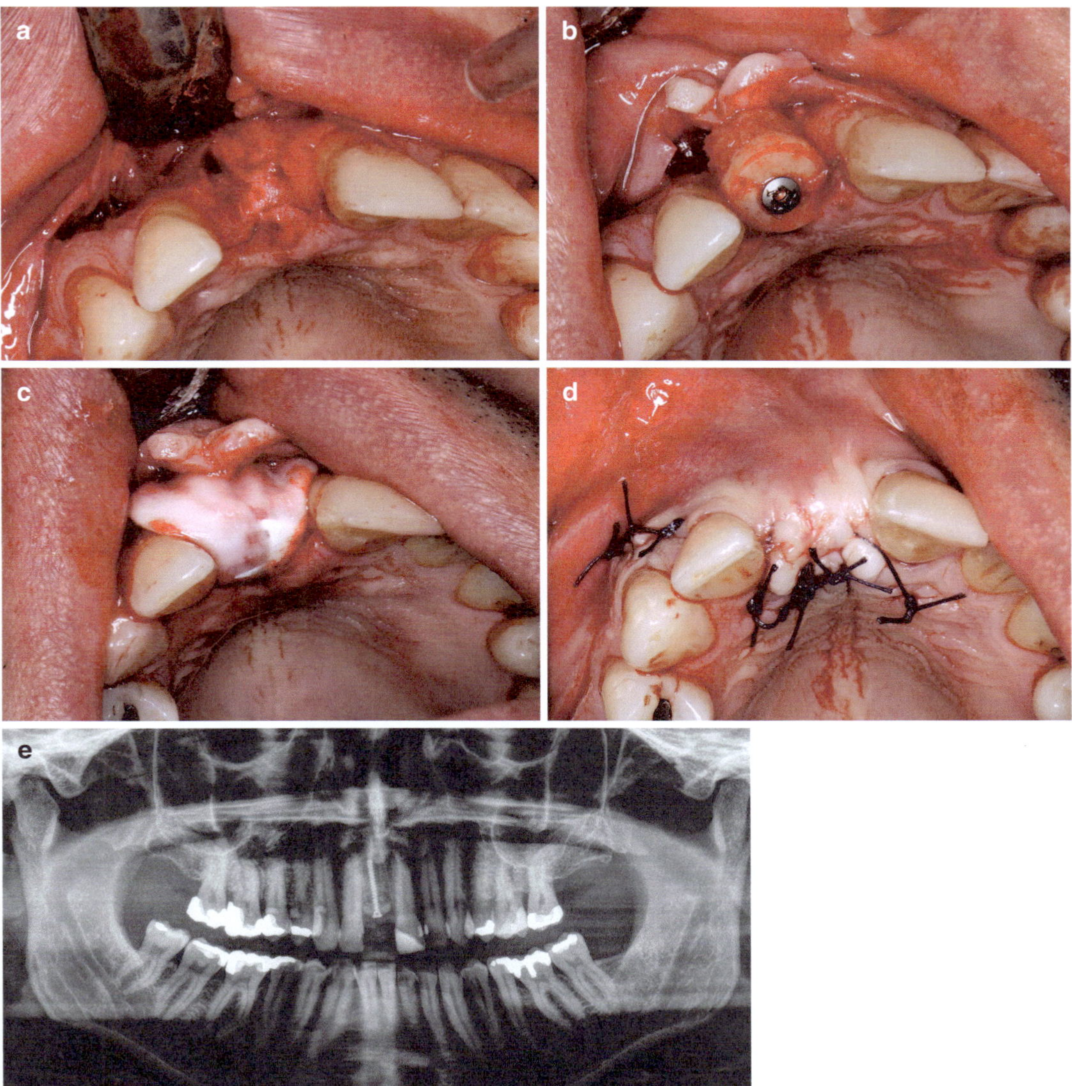

Fig. 8.9 (**a–e**) Here, the autologous cortical bone block was harvested at the mentum region. The bone block was fixed using an osteosynthesis screw. (© Karl Andreas Schlegel 2021. All Rights Reserved)

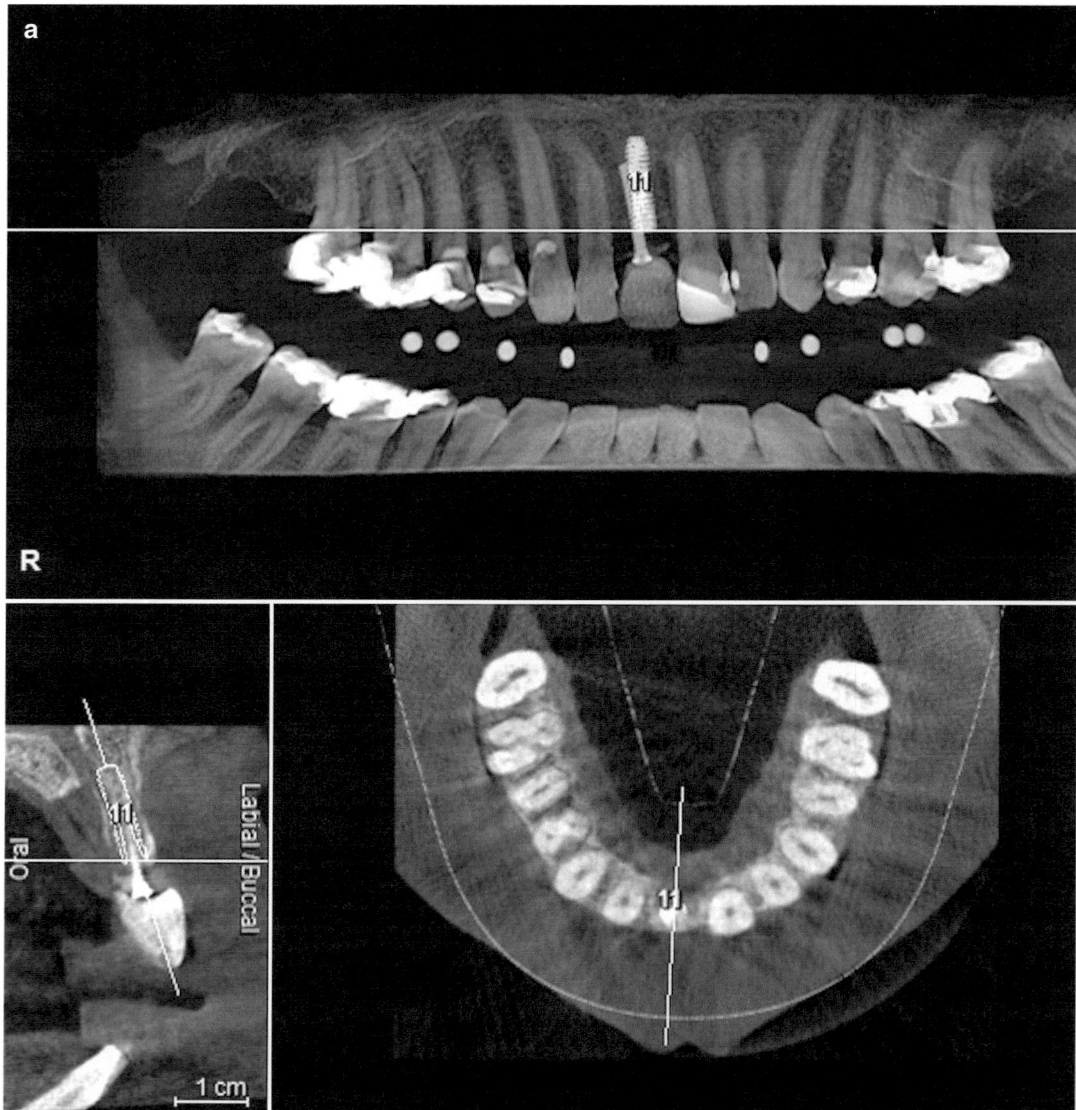

Fig. 8.10 (**a–c**) After the guided planning, the tooth-supported splint was fabricated in a dental laboratory. (© Karl Andreas Schlegel 2021. All Rights Reserved)

Implantat 11

b	Okklusaler Durchmesser	3.3 mm
	Apikaler Durchmesser	3.3 mm
	Länge	14 mm
	Hersteller	Straumann
	Implantatreihe	Bone Level Roxolid SLActive
	Seriennummer	021.2214

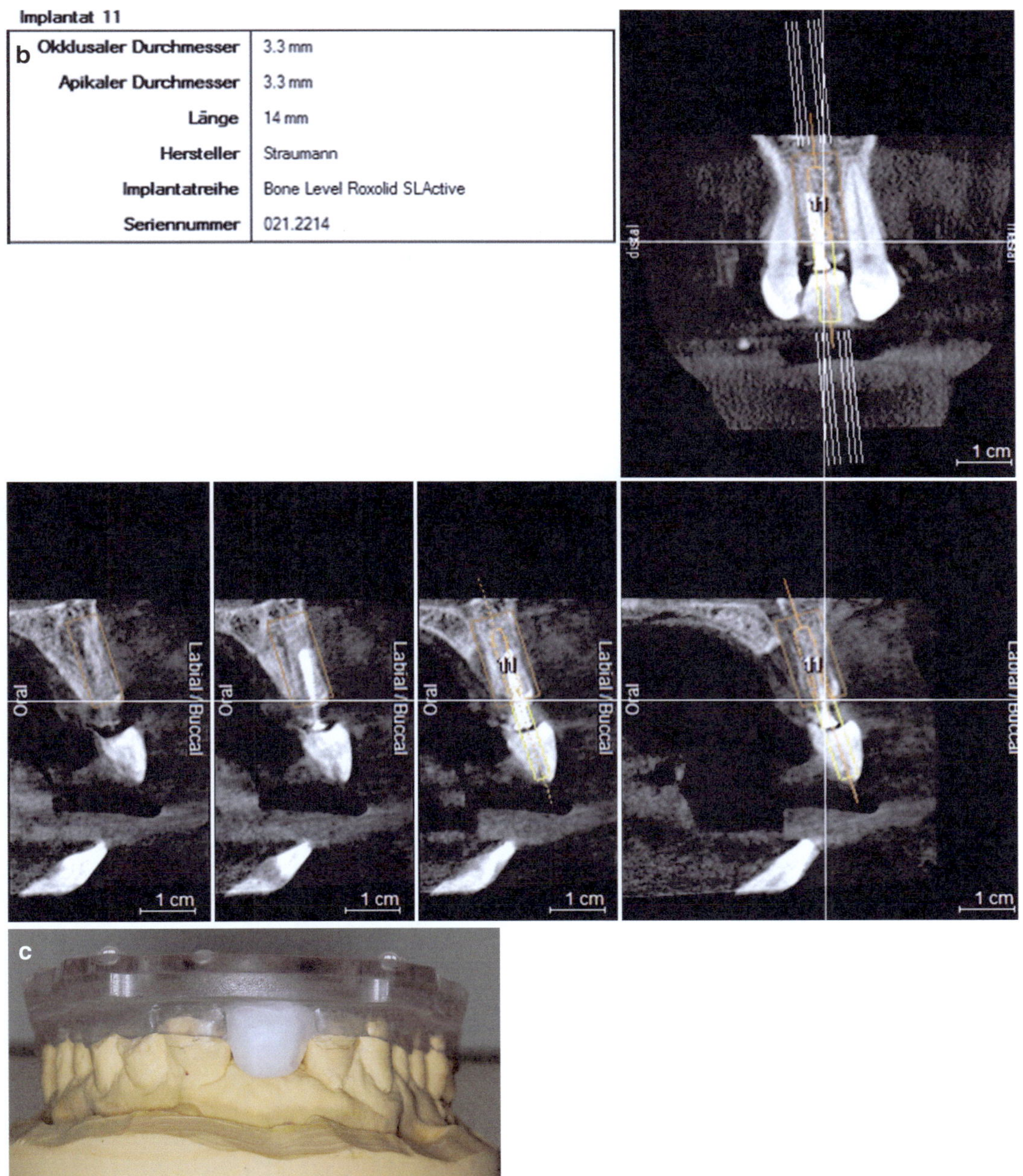

Fig. 8.10 (continued)

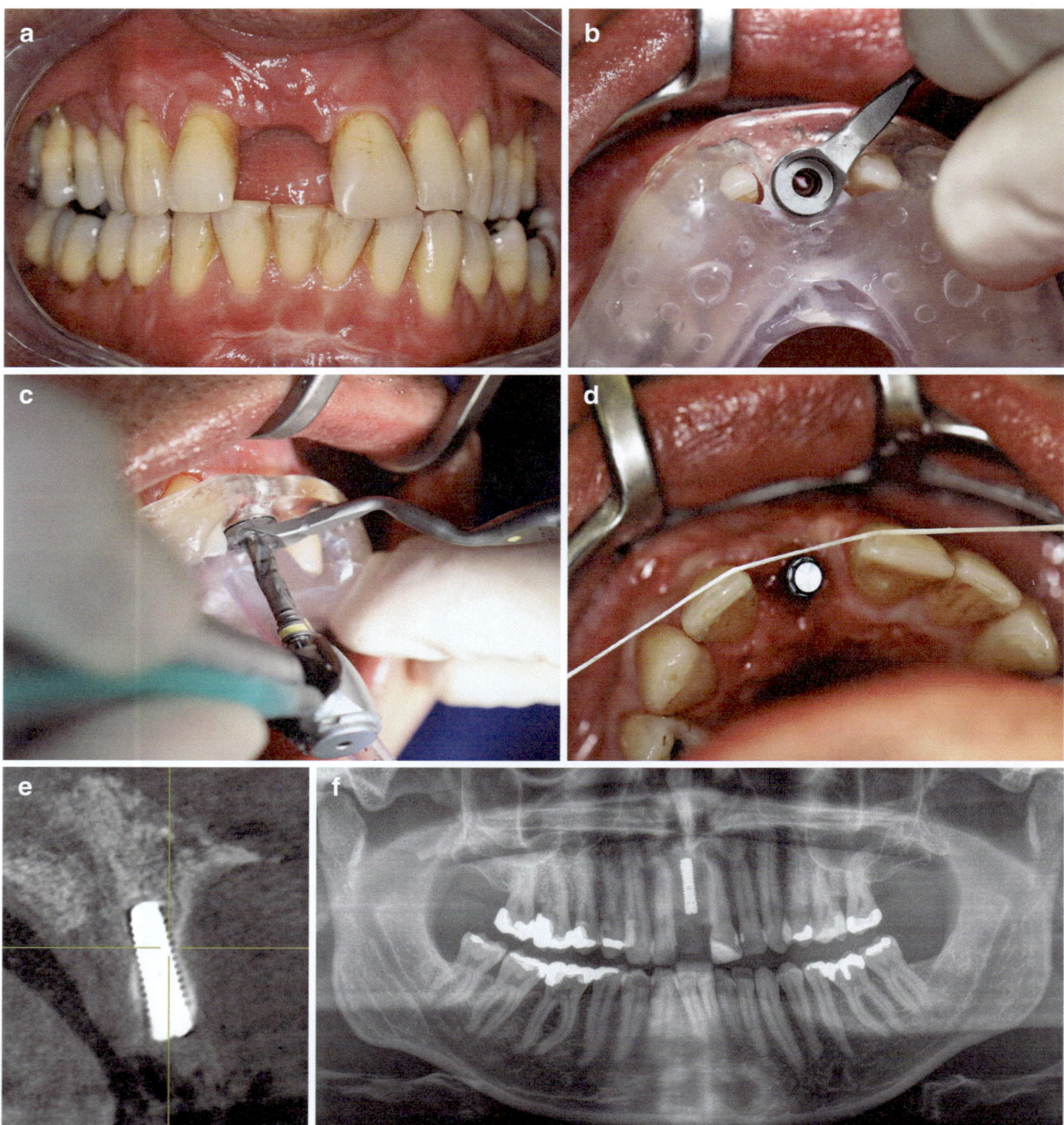

Fig. 8.11 (**a–f**) After optimal healing of the augmentation, the primary stable insertion of the implant took place. In (**e**), the narrow limits of anterior tooth implantation become apparent. (© Karl Andreas Schlegel 2021. All Rights Reserved)

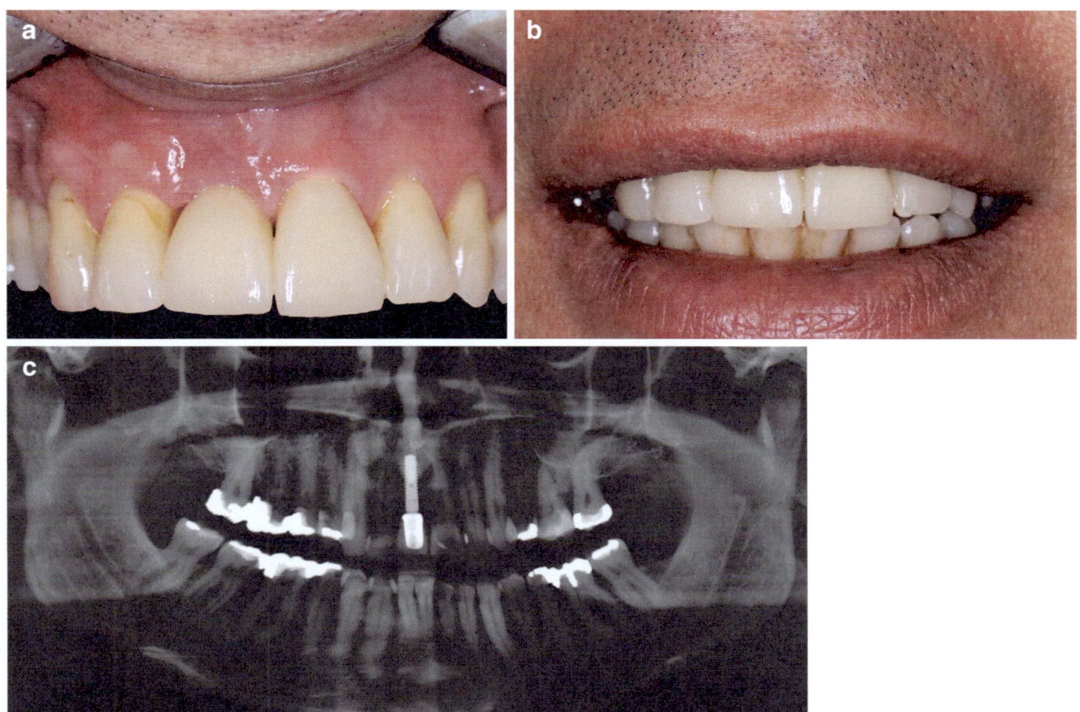

Fig. 8.12 (**a–c**) Six months after the referring colleague performed the final crown placement, this clinical and radiological follow-up took place. (© Karl Andreas Schlegel 2021. All Rights Reserved)

Guided Surgery with Temporary Implant-Supported Templates: Clinical Cases

9.1 Case I: Flapless (Figs. 9.1, 9.2, 9.3, 9.4, 9.5, 9.6, 9.7 and 9.8)

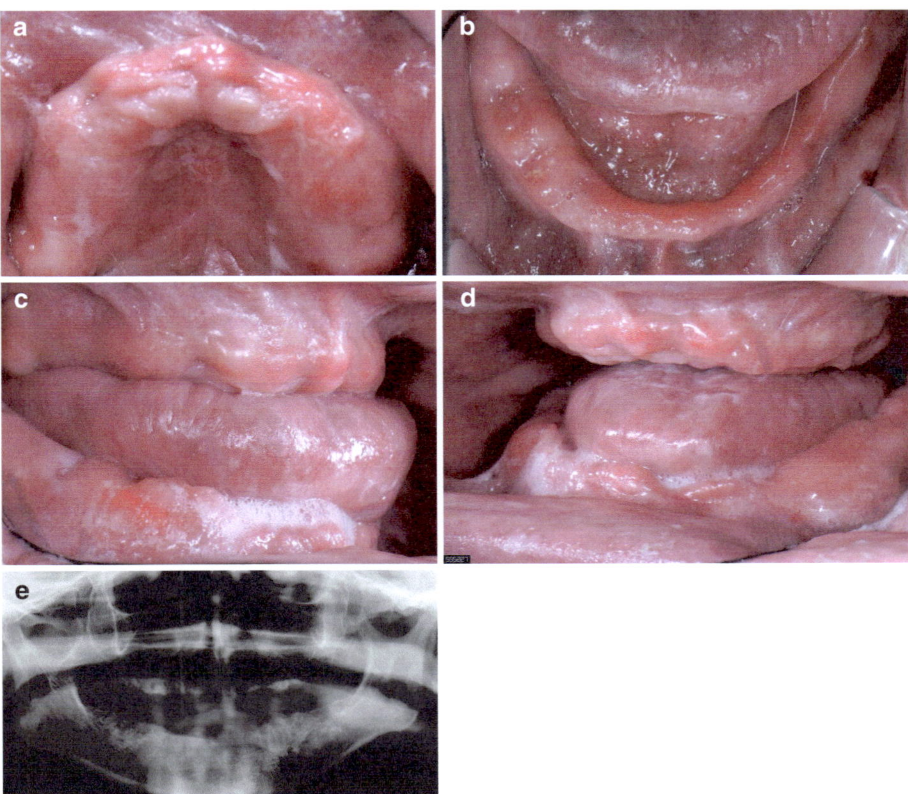

Fig. 9.1 (a–e) Especially in the mandible, the suction effect of the removable dentures is often insufficient due to bone atrophy, which is why many patients desire implant-supported anchorage. (© Karl Andreas Schlegel 2021. All Rights Reserved)

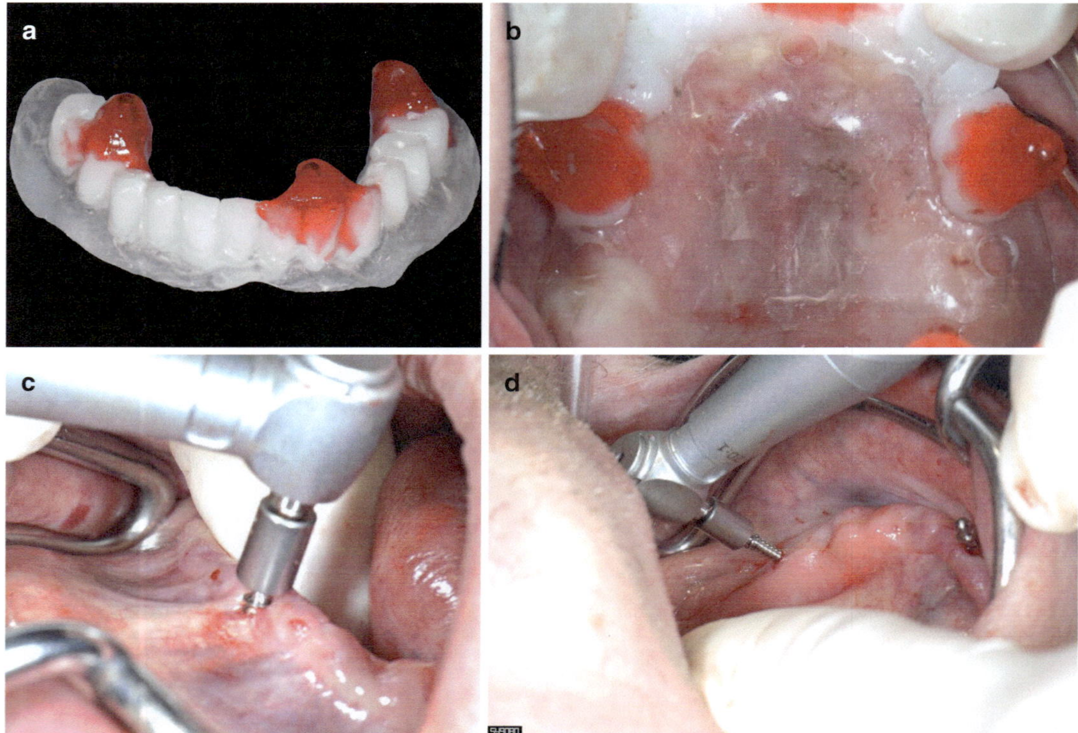

Fig. 9.2 (**a–d**) Gingiva-borne templates show greater inaccuracy when compared to tooth-supported templates due to the mobility of the mucosa. To increase accuracy, temporary implants may be used (e.g., in the case of a flabby ridge). (© Karl Andreas Schlegel 2021. All Rights Reserved)

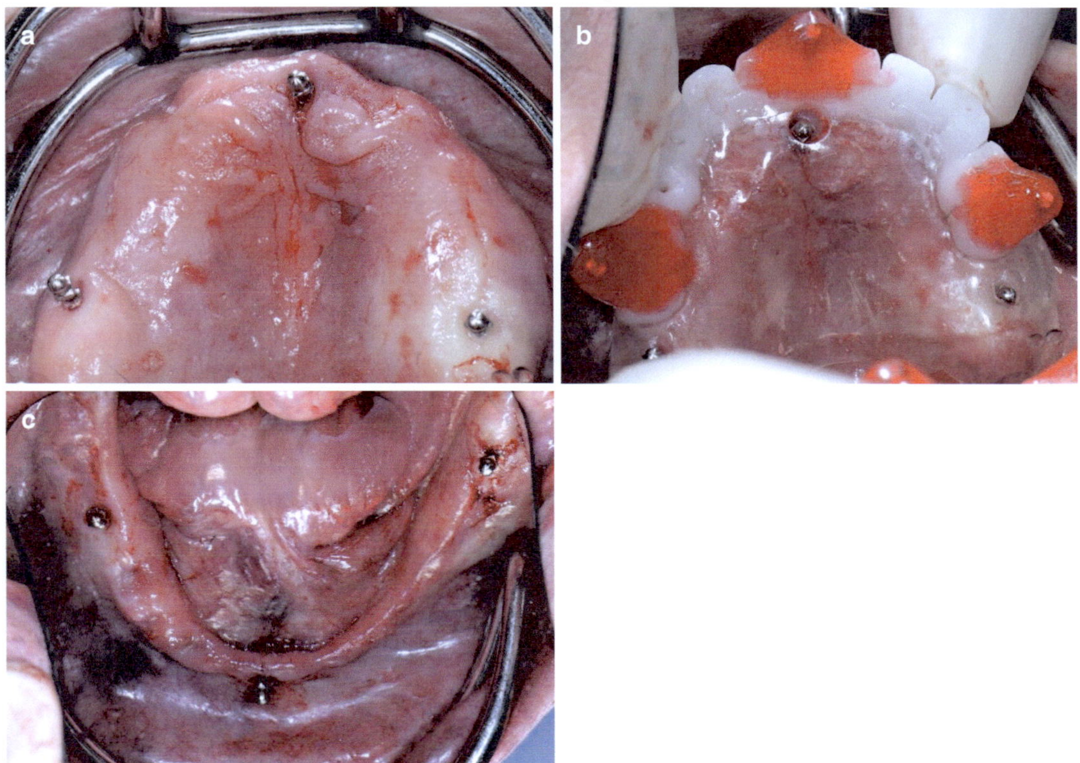

Fig. 9.3 (**a–c**) The temporary implants led to correct and reproducible template positioning. In order to avoid vertical deviations, vertical support using implants would also be conceivable. (© Karl Andreas Schlegel 2021. All Rights Reserved)

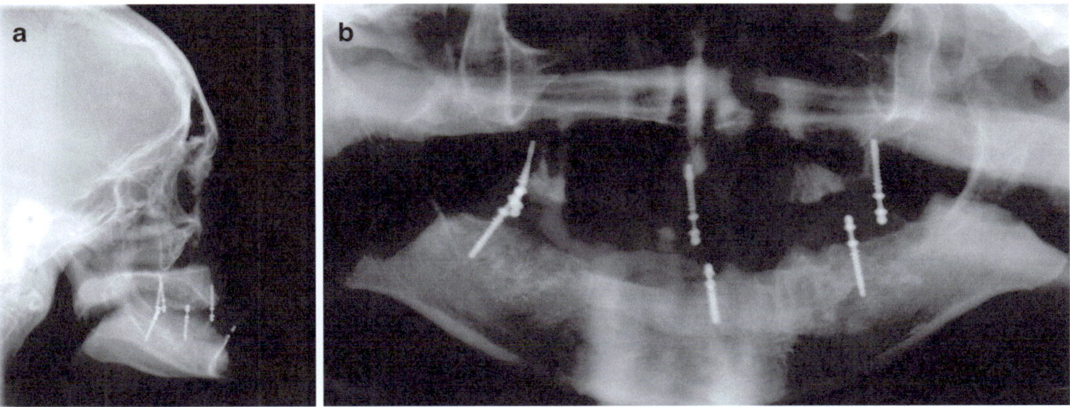

Fig. 9.4 (**a**, **b**) X-rays after the placement of the temporary implants. (© Karl Andreas Schlegel 2021. All Rights Reserved)

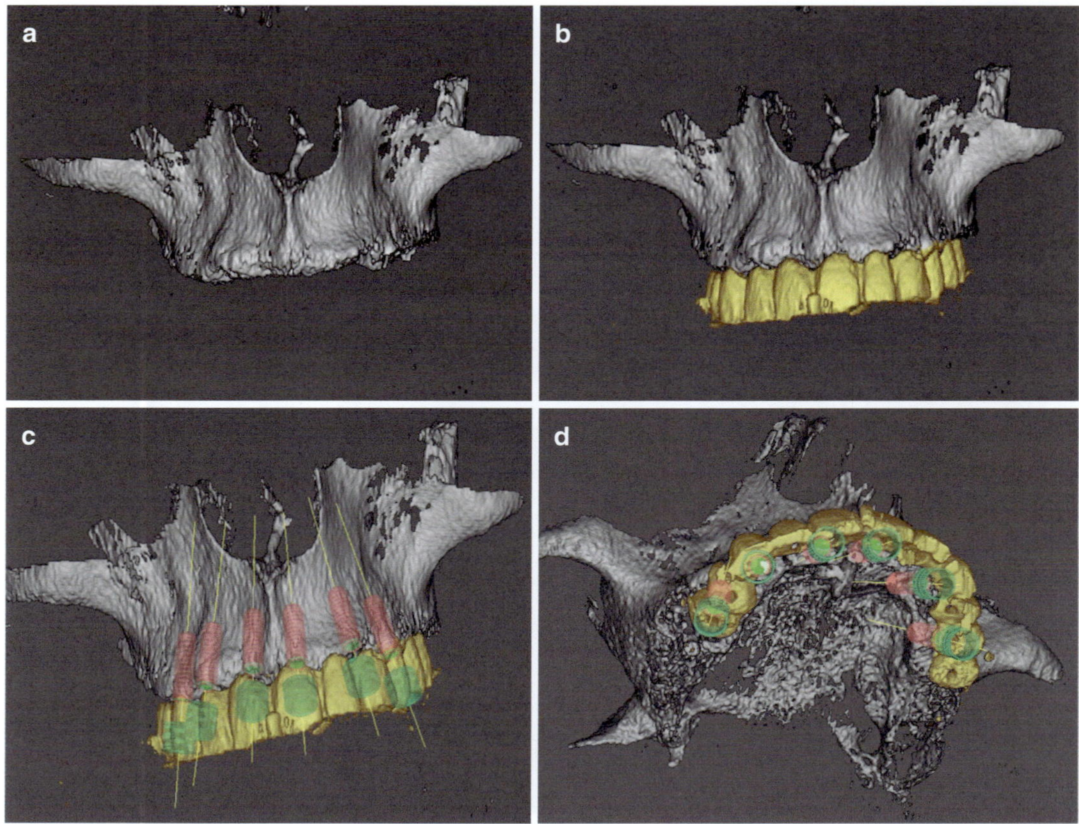

Fig. 9.5 (**a–d**) Segmentation and data matching for the upper jaw were presented before the planning of six implants. (© Karl Andreas Schlegel 2021. All Rights Reserved)

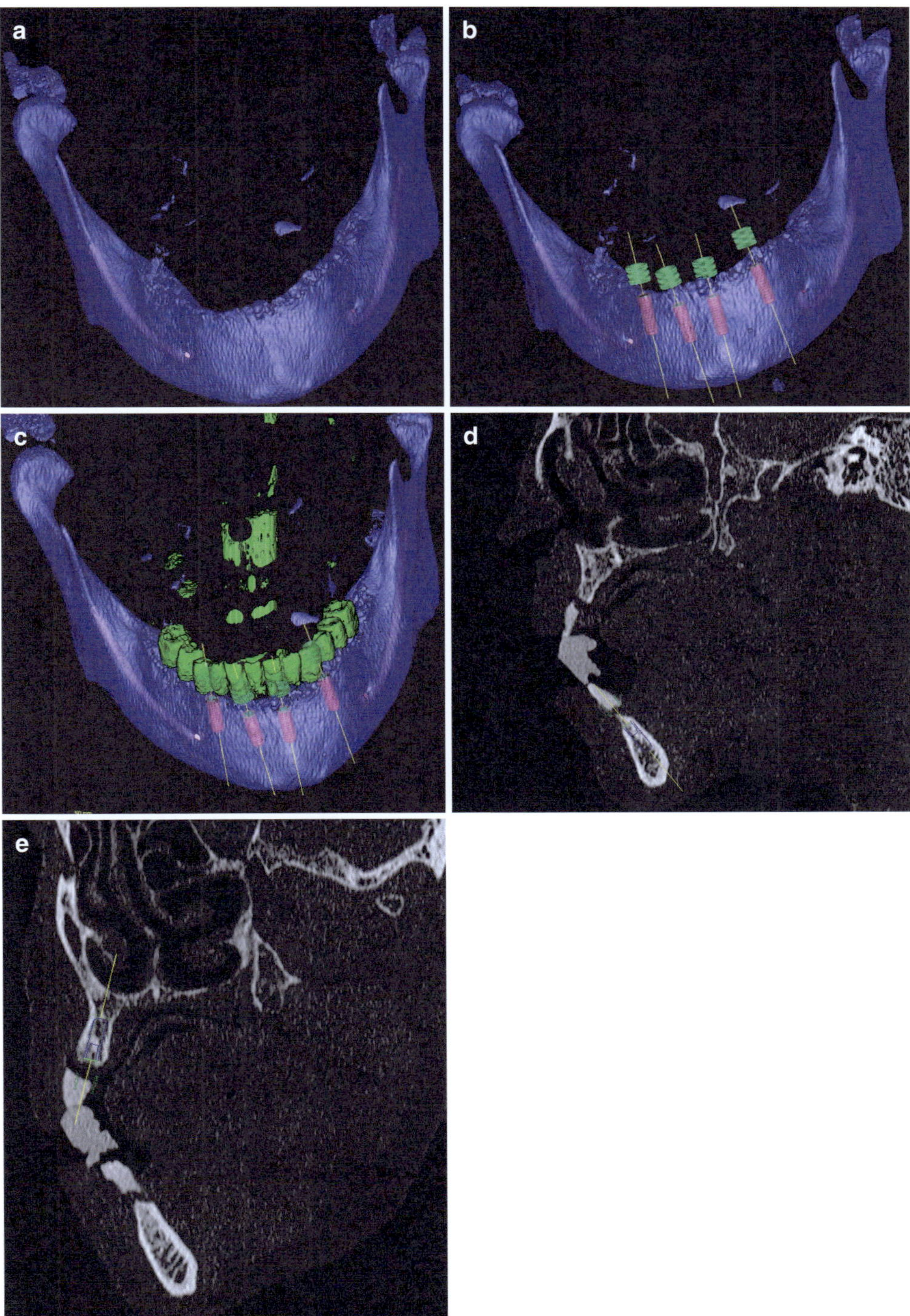

Fig. 9.6 (**a–g**) Segmentation and data matching were presented for the lower jaw before the planning of four implants. Finally, the software provided the drilling sequence (**f, g**). (© Karl Andreas Schlegel 2021. All Rights Reserved)

f

Farbkodierung	Position	Implantat-Art.-Nr.	Implantat	Hülse	Hülsenposition	Geführter Bohrer	Bohrlöffel	Planfräser
	15	021.4112 / G	SLActive Bone Level (Regular CrossFit™) Ø 4.1 mm 12 mm	H: 5 mm Ø: 5 mm	H4	≡ extra lang	●●● +3 mm	3.5 mm
	13	021.4112 / G	SLActive Bone Level (Regular CrossFit™) Ø 4.1 mm 12 mm	H: 5 mm Ø: 5 mm	H4	≡ extra lang	●●● +3 mm	3.5 mm
	11	021.4112 / G	SLActive Bone Level (Regular CrossFit™) Ø 4.1 mm 12 mm	H: 5 mm Ø: 5 mm	H4	≡ extra lang	●●● +3 mm	3.5 mm
	21	021.4112 / G	SLActive Bone Level (Regular CrossFit™) Ø 4.1 mm 12 mm	H: 5 mm Ø: 5 mm	H4	≡ extra lang	●●● +3 mm	3.5 mm
	23	021.4112 / G	SLActive Bone Level (Regular CrossFit™) Ø 4.1 mm 12 mm	H: 5 mm Ø: 5 mm	H4	≡ extra lang	●●● +3 mm	3.5 mm
	25	021.4112 / G	SLActive Bone Level (Regular CrossFit™) Ø 4.1 mm 12 mm	H: 5 mm Ø: 5 mm	H4	≡ extra lang	●●● +3 mm	3.5 mm

g

Farbkodierung	Position	Implantat-Art.-Nr.	Implantat	Hülse	Hülsenposition	Geführter Bohrer	Bohrlöffel	Planfräser
	44	021.4112 / G	SLActive Bone Level (Regular CrossFit™) Ø 4.1 mm 12 mm	H: 5 mm Ø: 5 mm	H6	≡ extra lang	●●● +3 mm	3.5 mm
	42	021.4112 / G	SLActive Bone Level (Regular CrossFit™) Ø 4.1 mm 12 mm	H: 5 mm Ø: 5 mm	H6	≡ extra lang	●●● +3 mm	3.5 mm
	32	021.4112 / G	SLActive Bone Level (Regular CrossFit™) Ø 4.1 mm 12 mm	H: 5 mm Ø: 5 mm	H6	≡ extra lang	●●● +3 mm	3.5 mm
	34	021.4112 / G	SLActive Bone Level (Regular CrossFit™) Ø 4.1 mm 12 mm	H: 5 mm Ø: 5 mm	H6	≡ extra lang	●●● +3 mm	3.5 mm

Fig. 9.6 (continued)

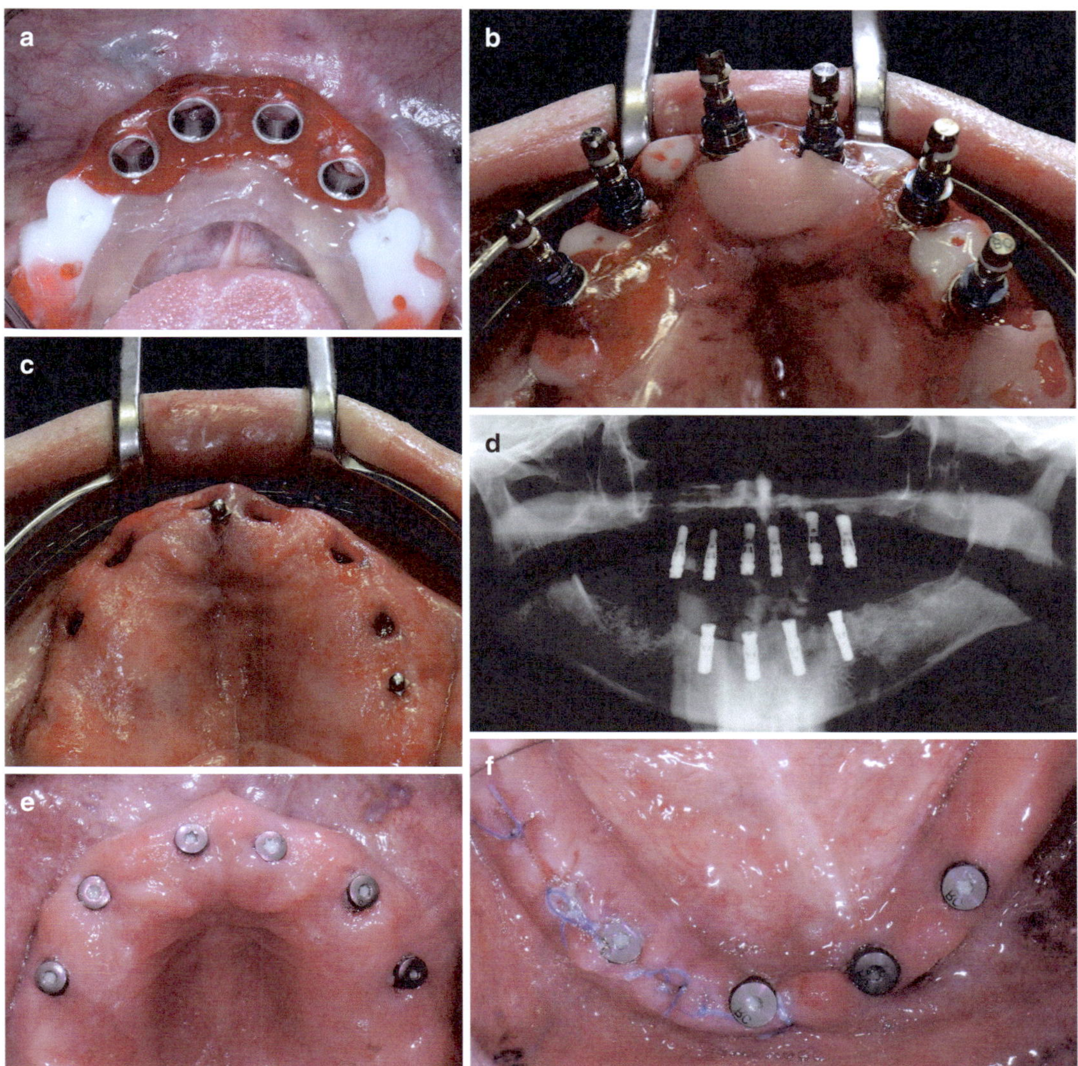

Fig. 9.7 (**a–f**) According to the full-guided planning, all ten implants were successfully placed. (© Karl Andreas Schlegel 2021. All Rights Reserved)

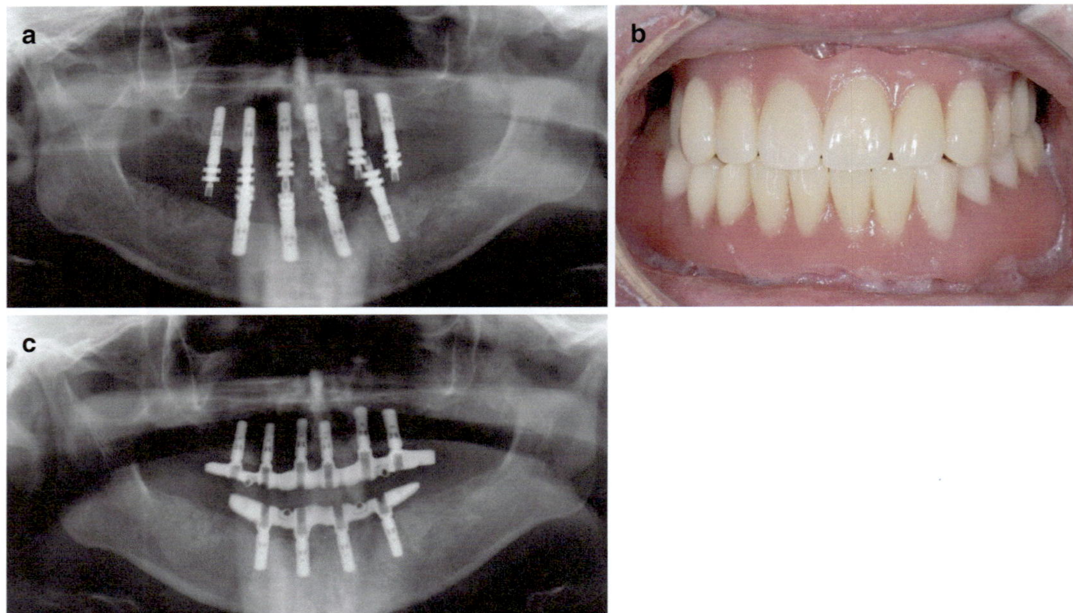

Fig. 9.8 (**a–c**) After the implant impression was taken, a bar anchorage was selected in the upper and lower jaws. (© Karl Andreas Schlegel 2021. All Rights Reserved)

Guided Surgery with Soft Tissue-Supported Templates: Clinical Cases

10.1 Case I: Flapless (Figs. 10.1, 10.2, 10.3, and 10.4)

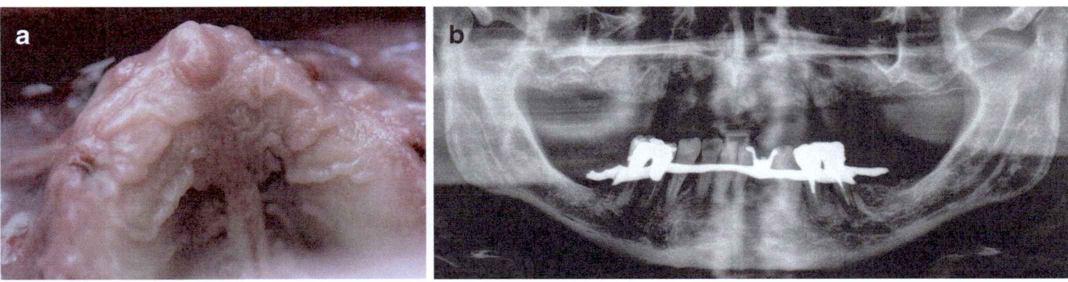

Fig. 10.1 (**a–b**) After the remaining maxillary teeth had to be extracted, the patient's wish was for an implant-supported removable maxillary prosthesis. (© Karl Andreas Schlegel 2021. All Rights Reserved)

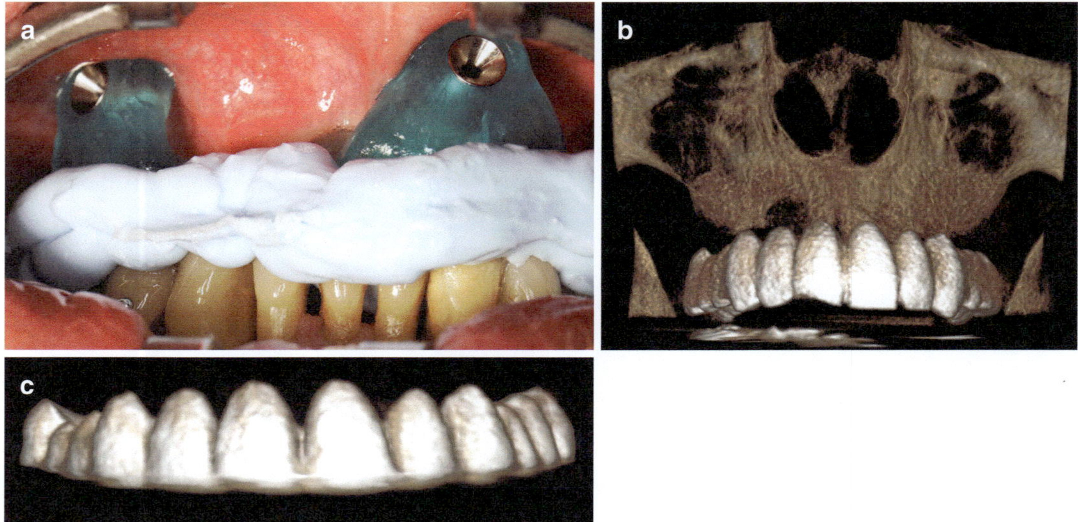

Fig. 10.2 (**a–c**) In this case, we used a double-scan technique, in which a CBCT scan was performed with the occlusion-secured template. Subsequently, the template alone was scanned and then matched. (© Karl Andreas Schlegel 2021. All Rights Reserved)

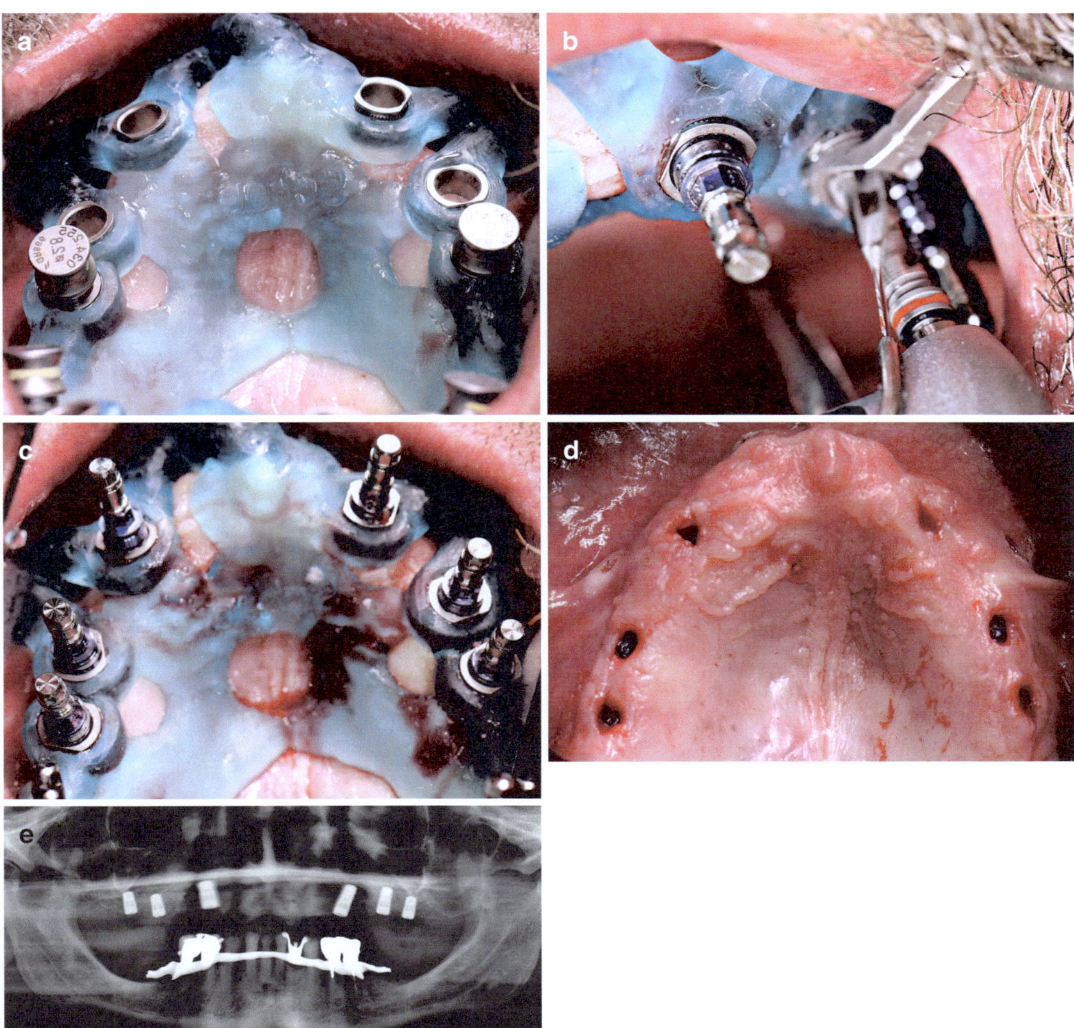

Fig. 10.3 (**a–e**) After the digital planning and positioning of six implants, guided implant placement was performed with a gingiva-borne template and a flapless approach. (© Karl Andreas Schlegel 2021. All Rights Reserved)

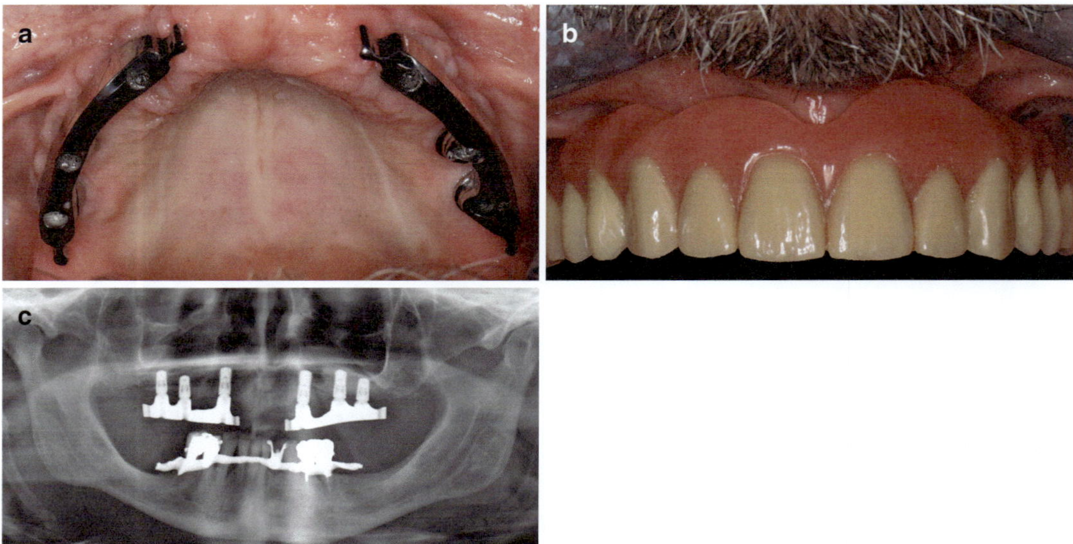

Fig. 10.4 (**a–c**) The smile line and the level of the crestal bone in the maxilla led to the recommendation of a removable prosthesis with a labial flange in this case. The 1-year follow-up is shown here. (© Karl Andreas Schlegel 2021. All Rights Reserved)

10.2 **Case II: With Flap** (Figs. 10.5, 10.6, 10.7, 10.8, 10.9, and 10.10)

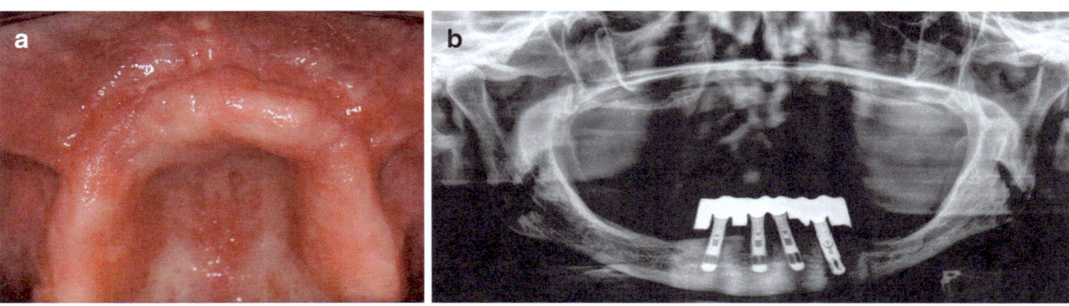

Fig. 10.5 (**a**, **b**) The patient's lower jaw had already been restored using four implants and a removable denture. An implant-supported denture for the upper jaw was also planned to be fabricated. However, there was a pronounced bone deficit. (© Karl Andreas Schlegel 2021. All Rights Reserved)

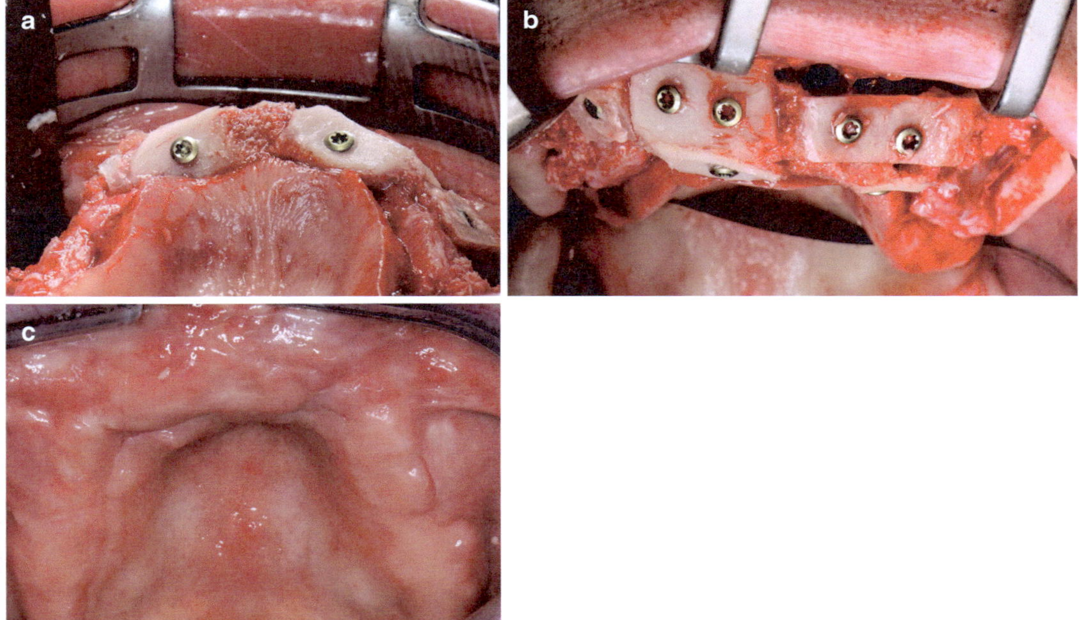

Fig. 10.6 (**a–c**) In order to achieve the necessary bone volume, cortical bone augmentation from the iliac crest was planned in this case. (© Karl Andreas Schlegel 2021. All Rights Reserved)

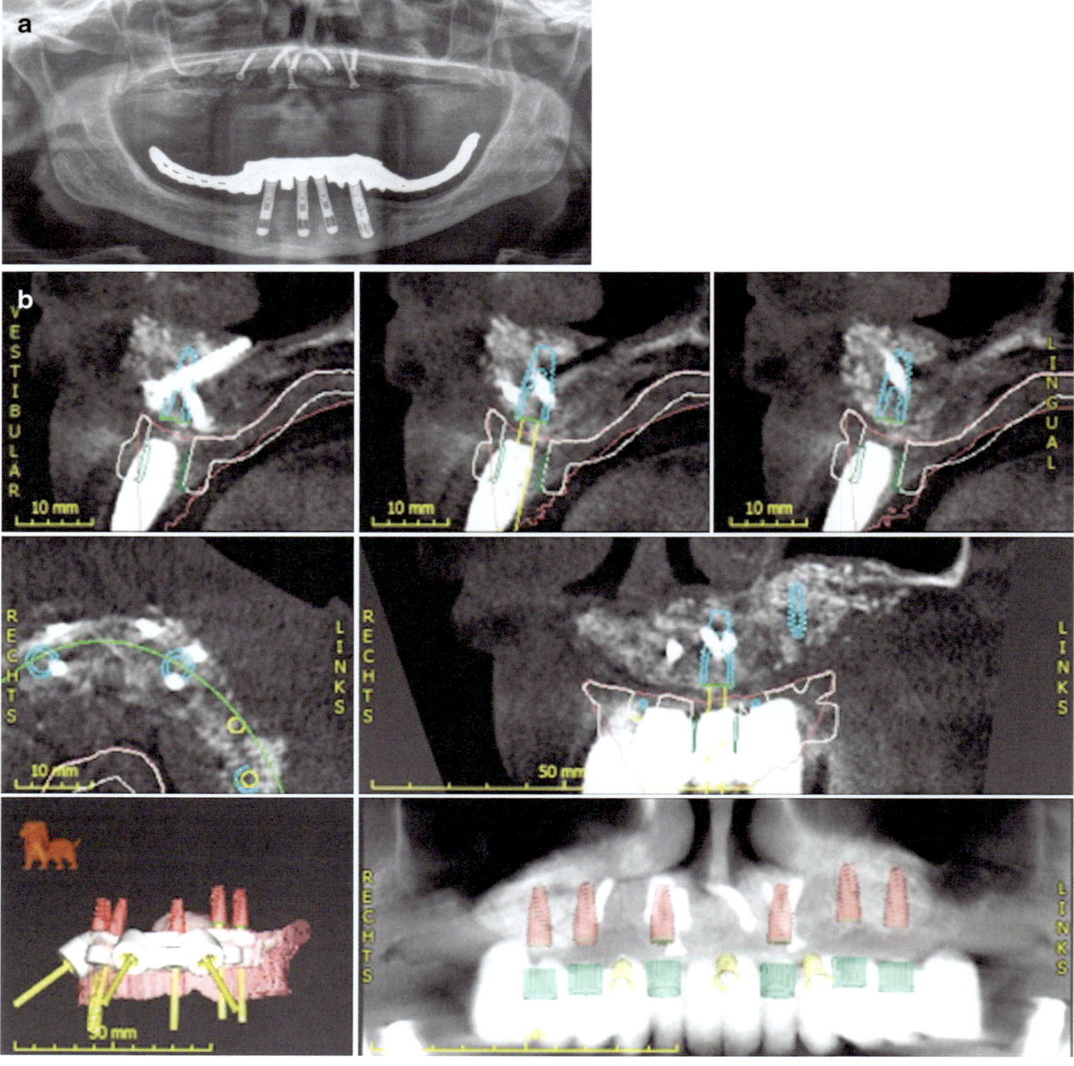

Fig. 10.7 (**a**, **b**) After a sufficient healing period of 4 months, three-dimensional imaging and subsequent full-guided planning were performed. (© Karl Andreas Schlegel 2021. All Rights Reserved)

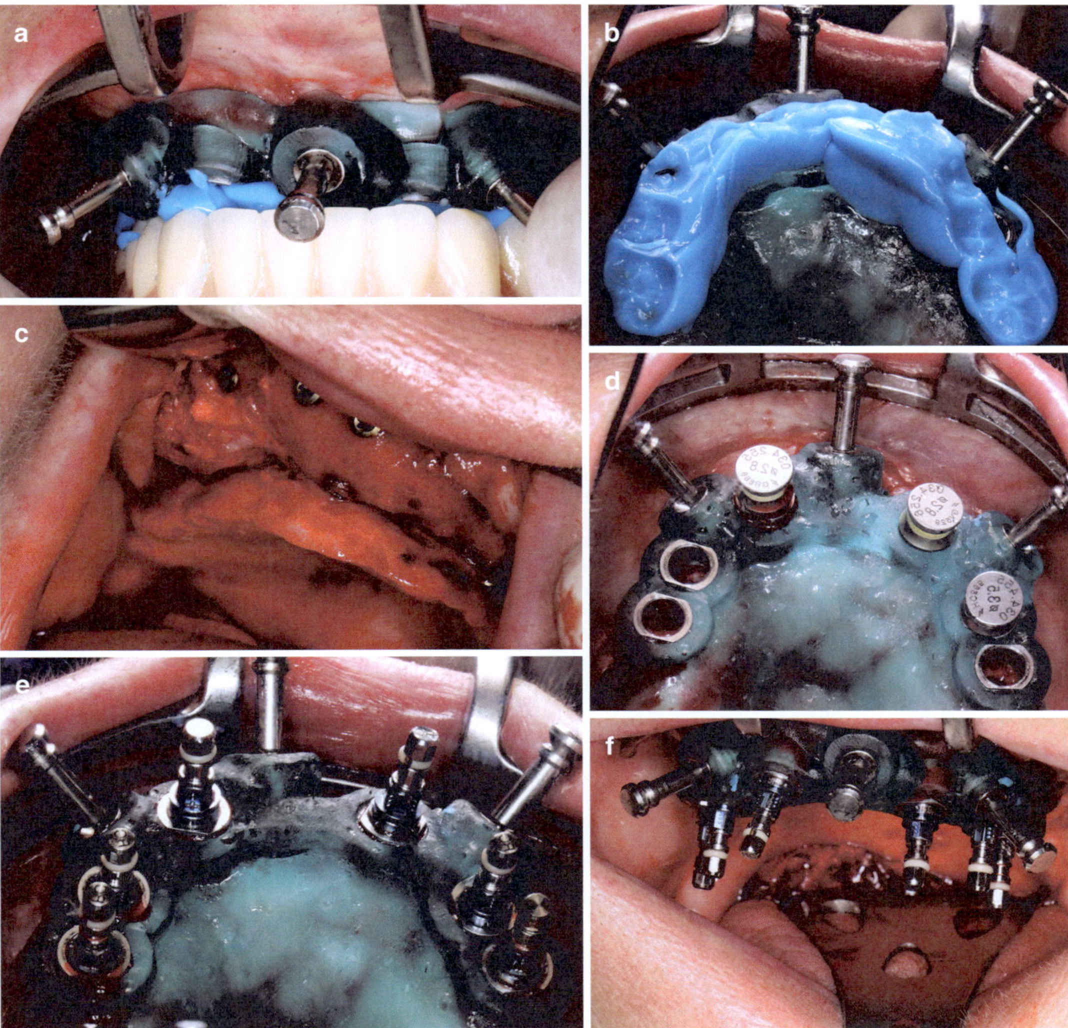

Fig. 10.8 (**a**, **b**) Due to soft tissue mobility, the gingiva-borne template was kept in position with the interdental occlusion not only during imaging but also during surgery to insert the positioning screws. (**c–f**) The augmented bone proved to be volume stable, and after the fixation of the template, all implants could be inserted according to the drill sequence. (© Karl Andreas Schlegel 2021. All Rights Reserved)

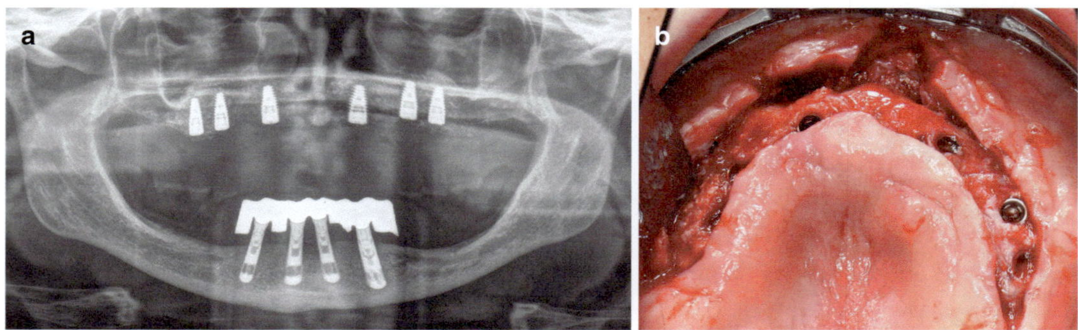

Fig. 10.9 (**a**, **b**) Over the 3-month healing phase of the implants, stable hard and soft tissue conditions were revealed during implant exposure. (© Karl Andreas Schlegel 2021. All Rights Reserved)

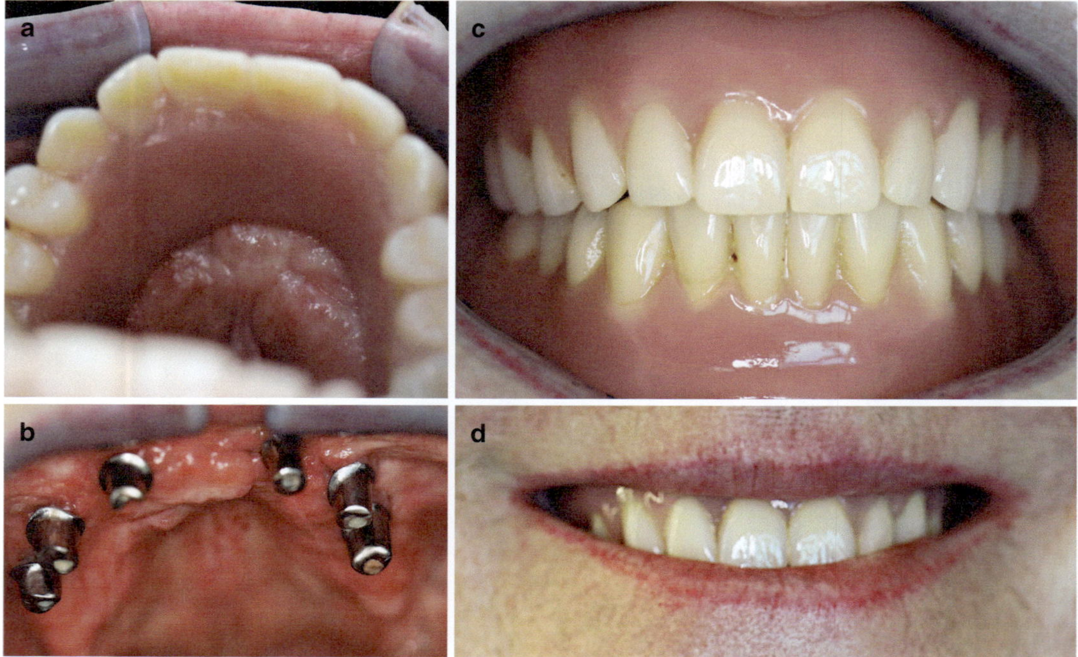

Fig. 10.10 (**a–d**) To support the removable maxillary prosthesis, telescopic crowns were selected as anchorage elements. The advantage of this restoration was the labial flange of the prosthesis, which could ideally define the smile line and upper lip profile. (© Karl Andreas Schlegel 2021. All Rights Reserved)

10.3 Case III: With Flap (Figs. 10.11, 10.12, 10.13, 10.14, 10.15, and 10.16)

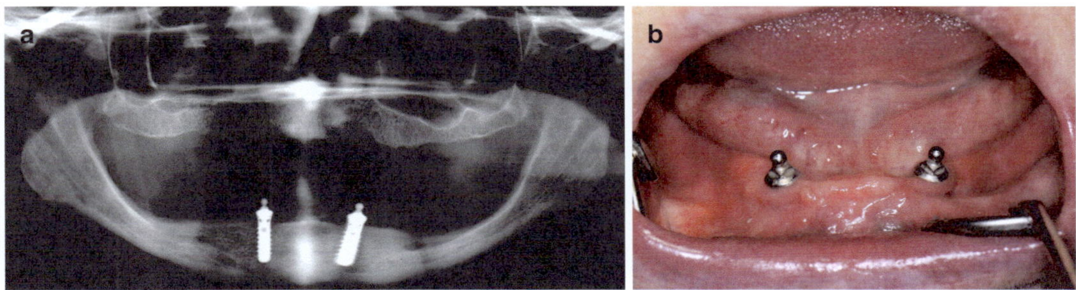

Fig. 10.11 (**a**, **b**) The initial situation included an edentulous maxilla and two implants in the mandible. (© Karl Andreas Schlegel 2021. All Rights Reserved)

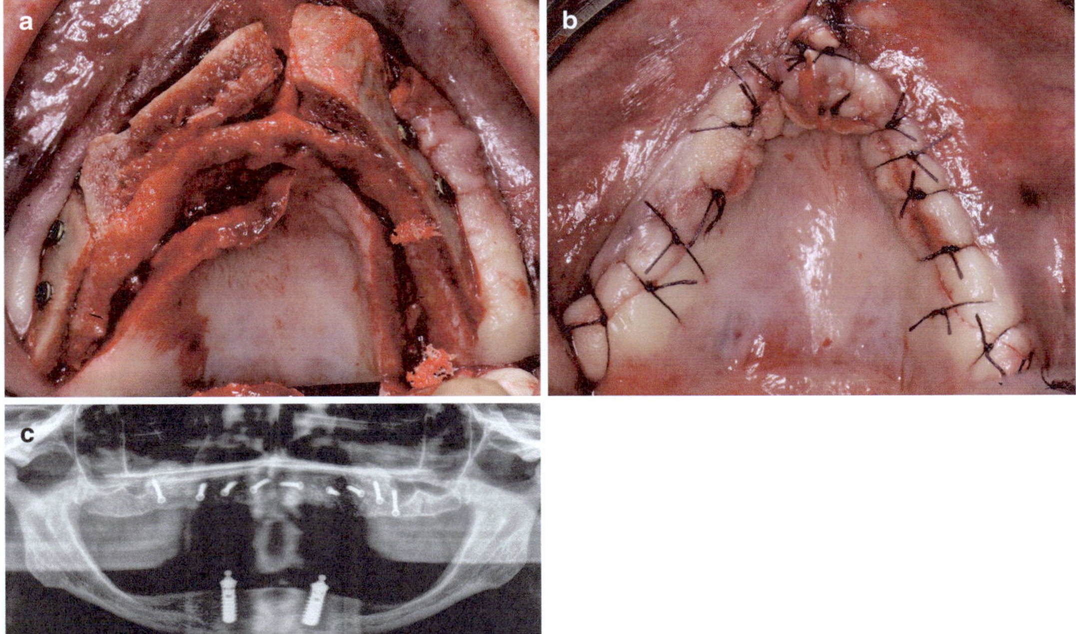

Fig. 10.12 (**a–c**) Due to bone atrophy, an augmentation with bone from the iliac crest had to be performed before the full-guided implant planning. (© Karl Andreas Schlegel 2021. All Rights Reserved)

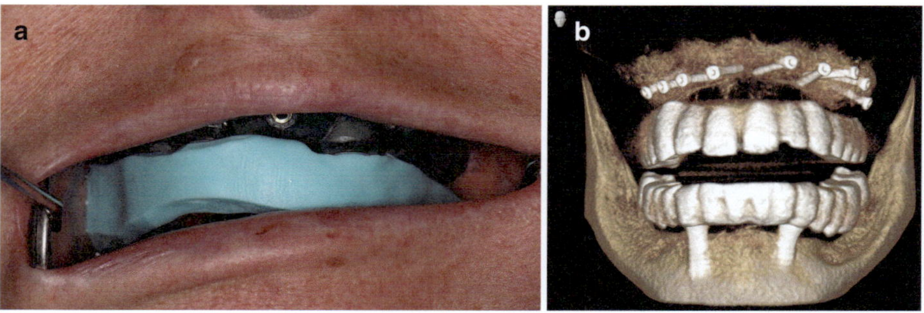

Fig. 10.13 (**a**, **b**) Due to soft tissue mobility, the gingiva-borne template was kept in position with the interdental occlusion during imaging. (© Karl Andreas Schlegel 2021. All Rights Reserved)

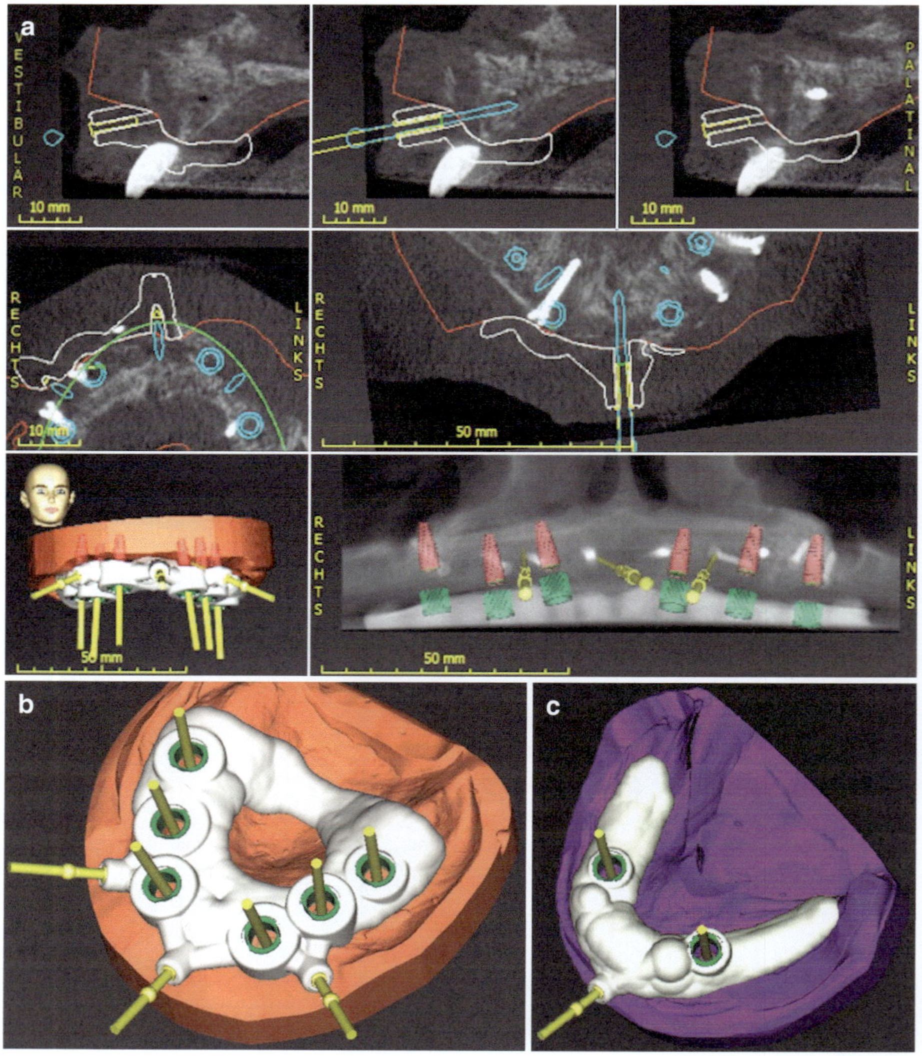

Fig. 10.14 (**a–c**) Full-guided implant positioning for both jaws in the planning software. (© Karl Andreas Schlegel 2021. All Rights Reserved)

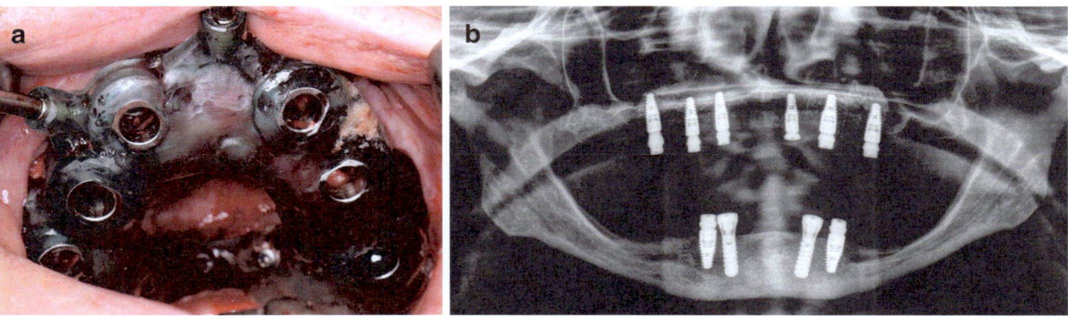

Fig. 10.15 (**a, b**) Full-guided implant surgery was performed in the upper and lower jaws. (© Karl Andreas Schlegel 2021. All Rights Reserved)

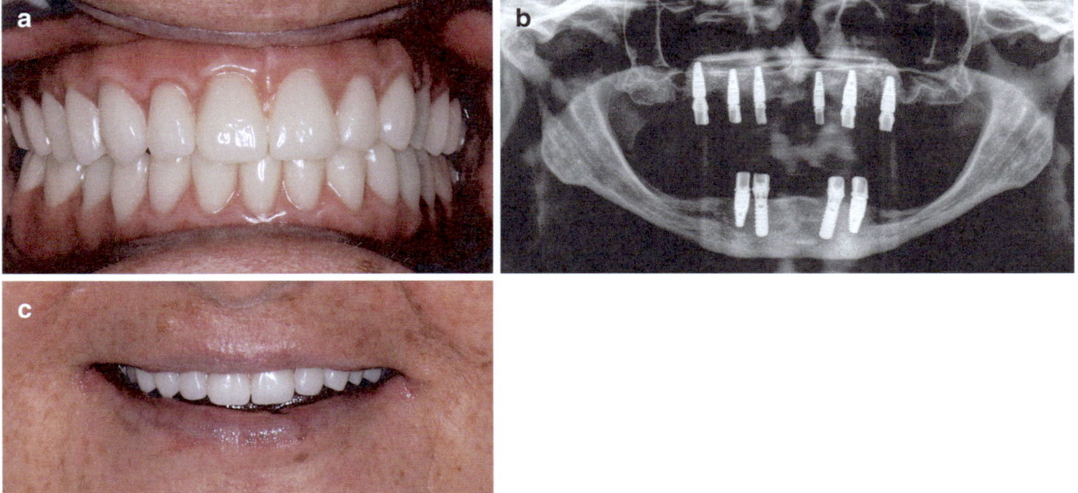

Fig. 10.16 (**a–c**) The final result after 1.5 years of follow-up. (© Karl Andreas Schlegel 2021. All Rights Reserved)

10.4   Case IV: With Flap (Figs. 10.17, 10.18, 10.19, 10.20, and 10.21)

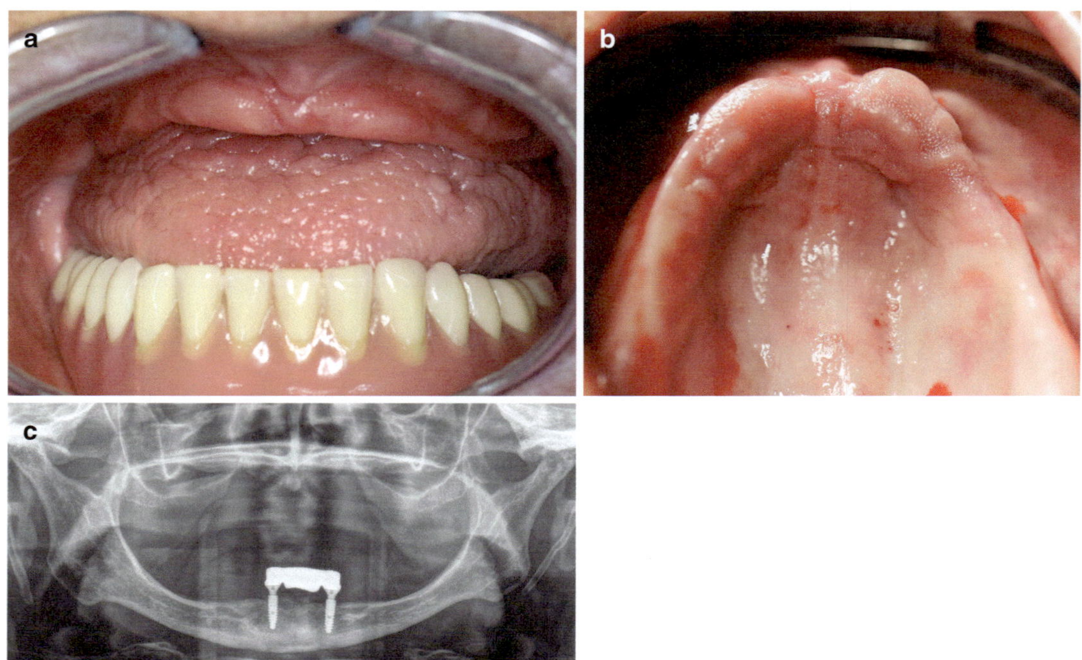

Fig. 10.17 (**a–c**) The initial situation included an edentulous maxilla and two implants in the mandible, again with severe atrophy. (© Karl Andreas Schlegel 2021. All Rights Reserved)

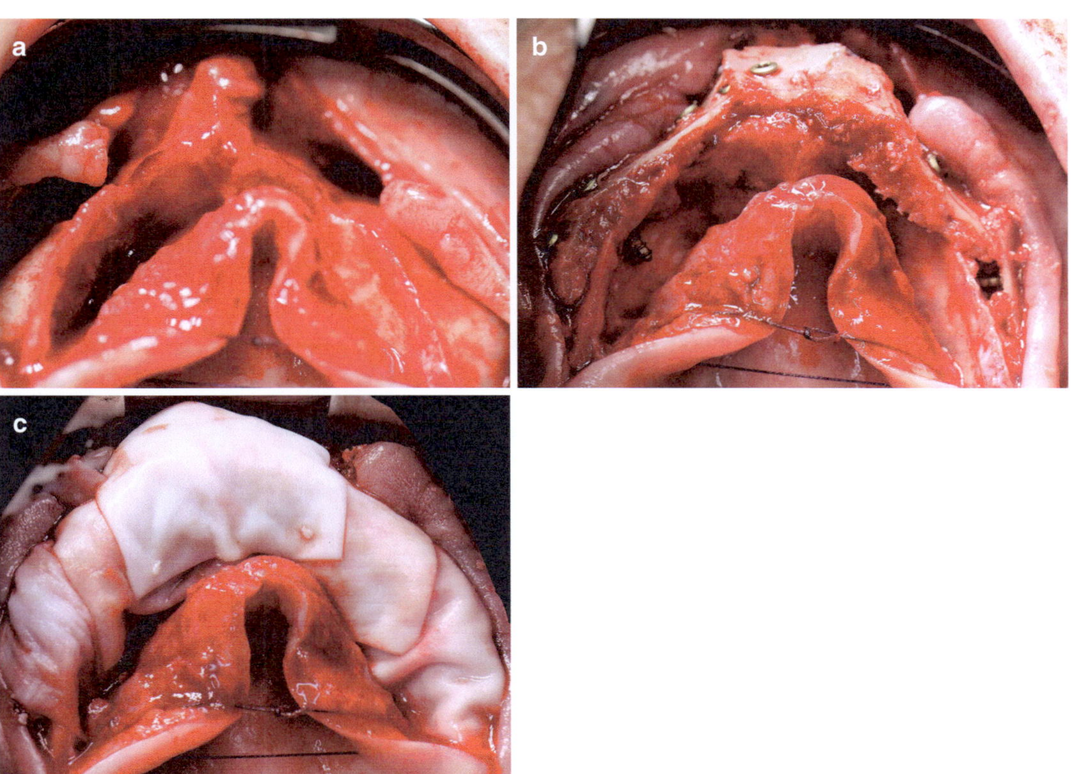

Fig. 10.18 (**a–c**) Augmentation with bone from the iliac crest was performed in the upper jaw before implant surgery. (© Karl Andreas Schlegel 2021. All Rights Reserved)

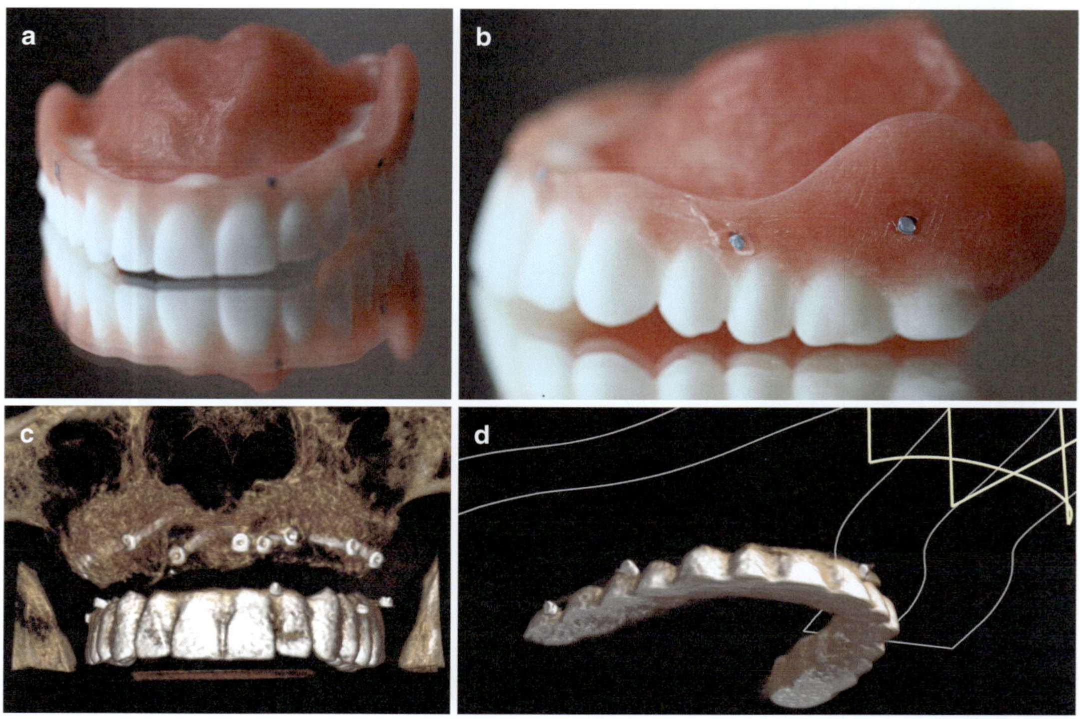

Fig. 10.19 (**a–d**) A double-scan technique was used, in which a CBCT scan was performed with the occlusion-secured template. Subsequently, the template alone was scanned using CBCT. Afterward, the two digital files could be matched in the software using the inserted reference points. (© Karl Andreas Schlegel 2021. All Rights Reserved)

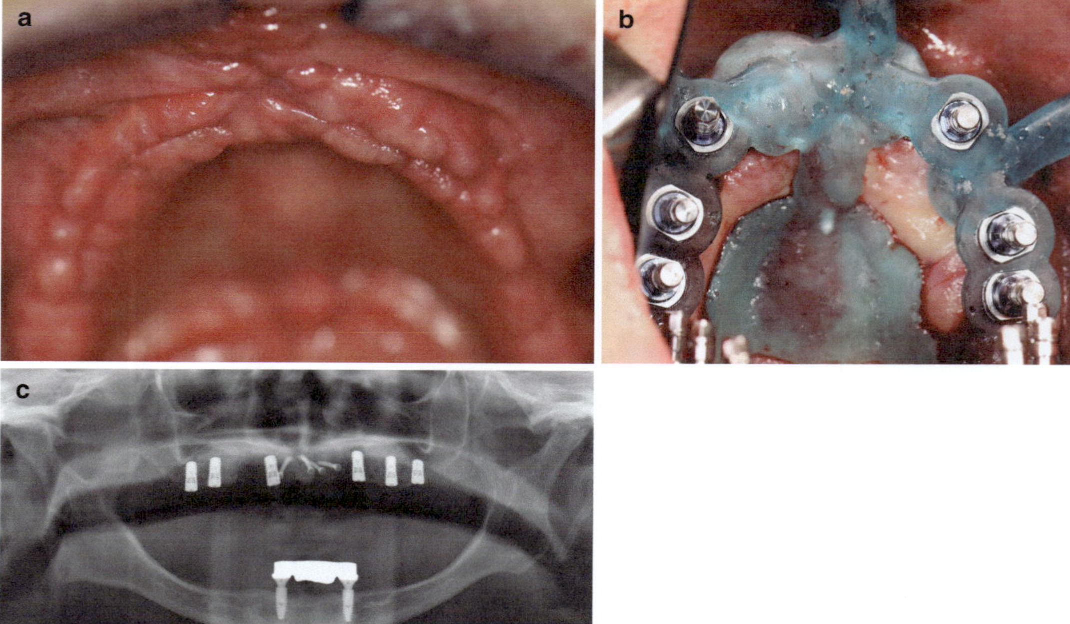

Fig. 10.20 (**a–c**) These pictures show the guided implant placement and the postoperative radiographic control image. (© Karl Andreas Schlegel 2021. All Rights Reserved)

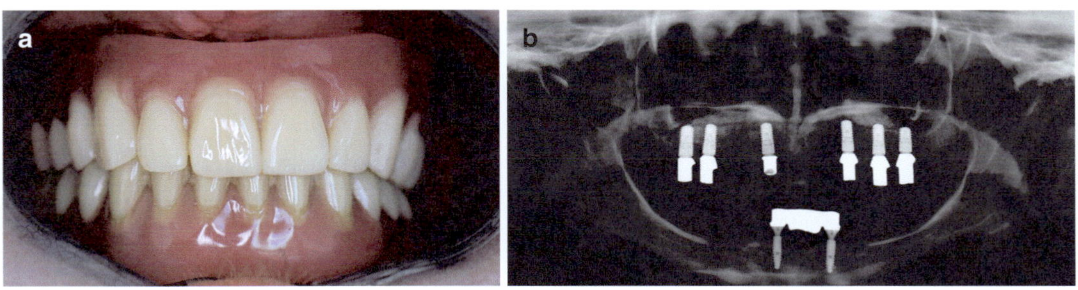

Fig. 10.21 (**a**, **b**) The final denture of the upper jaw was anchored using telescopic crowns. (© Karl Andreas Schlegel 2021. All Rights Reserved)

Learning Objective
- Are you familiar with the digital planning of a preoperative immediate provisional denture?

Patients often desire quick rather than complex and time-consuming solutions for their dental treatment. The unloaded healing phase of the implant body, especially in difficult cases, is the safest option for the highest possible integration rate [1]. A possible immediate restoration with a simultaneous reduction of appointments may considerably increase patient comfort [2]. Computer-guided surgery can significantly improve the predictability of the therapy and the comfort of the patient [3]. This can be achieved using, for example, concepts that use immediate loading of the implant bodies directly after implant placement [2]. Procedures may be combined with simultaneous extractions, immediate implant placement, and immediate loading or immediate restoration using a temporary denture. The prosthetic restoration can range from single-tooth crowns to full-arch restorations. If immediate implant loading is intended, one must consider the stability of the primary implant, the need for substantial bone augmentation, implant design and dimension, occlusal factors, patient habits, systemic health, and clinician experience [1]. This applies to protocols for single implants in partially edentulous patients and implant-supported overdentures in edentulous jaws as well. When initial implant loading is planned, the primary implant should have an insertion torque ≥ 30 Ncm and/or an implant stability quotient (ISQ) ≥ 60 [1].

Degidi and Piattelli showed that immediate functional restoration can present satisfactory results in selected cases [4, 5]. However, patients should be carefully selected for either immediate loading or immediate restoration. In cases with poor primary implant stability, substantial bone augmentation, implants of reduced dimensions, and compromised host conditions, in agreement with the fifth ITI Consensus Conference, a predictable conventional delayed implant loading should be preferred [1].

Conventionally, immediate implantological loading is achieved by means of an intraoperative impression and the subsequent fabrication of the work in the dental laboratory. Full-guided surgery offers the possibility of fabricating temporary dentures prior to surgery in order to provide immediate restoration of the implant bodies or even occlusal loading [6]. However, due to possible inaccuracies in the process, prefabrication of the final prosthetic restoration before surgery cannot be recommended [7].

In this concept, the implants are inserted through the drilling template with the appropriate alignment. After removal of the implant insertion aids and of the drilling template, the primary stability can be measured using, for example, the Osstell implant stability values

(W&H Dentalwerk GmbH, Bürmoos, Austria) [8]. The existing temporary denture was previously prepared in the dental laboratory, considering the implant positions. During the insertion of the prosthesis, the wound areas must be protected against excess pressing from the fluid materials. Subsequently, the individual abutments (prepared in advance) are inserted (Fig. 11.1).

Here, the denture is bonded to the abutments with light-curing resin. Furthermore, a relining impression can simultaneously be taken. In the dental laboratory, the manipulation implants are screwed onto the temporary abutments and incorporated into the existing model. The denture is then completed in the laboratory within a short time and can then be inserted intraorally.

Sufficient primary stability shortly after implant placement is essential to ensure that the restoration is placed in the mouth on the same day [1]. Excessive pressure on the soft tissue due to denture components must be avoided.

11.1 Conclusion

If immediate implant loading is intended, the primary implant stability should at least have an insertion torque ≥30 Ncm and/or an ISQ ≥60. Nevertheless, in cases with poor primary implant stability, substantial bone augmentation, implants of reduced dimensions, and compromised host conditions, predictable conventional delayed implant loading should be preferred.

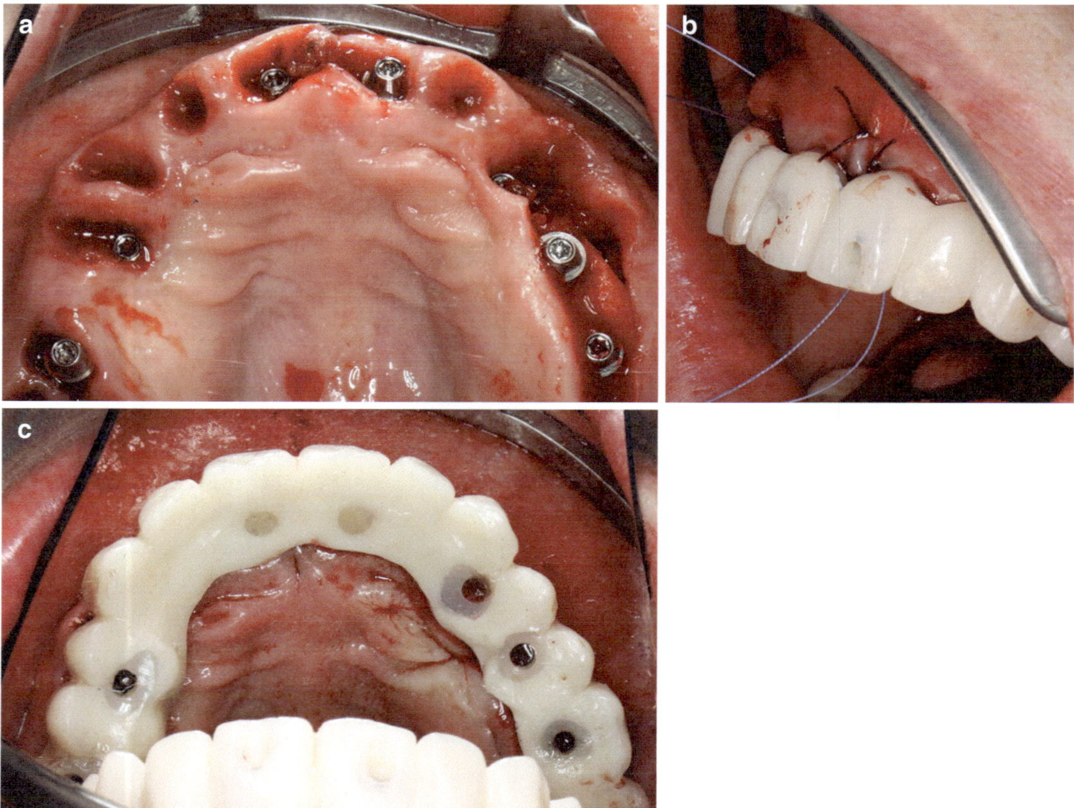

Fig. 11.1 (**a**) In this case, a full-guided implant placement with a subsequent immediate loading is presented. (**b**) The existing temporary denture was previously prepared in the dental laboratory and was inserted during surgery. The suturing of the wound was performed at the end. (**c**) Occlusal view of the screw-retained provisional denture in the maxilla. (© Andreas Schlegel 2021. All Rights Reserved)

A Clinical Case

Case I: Flapless

In rare cases and for a selection of patients, immediate implantation and immediate restoration may also be considered. In this case, the patient had chronic periodontitis. The condition was consistently treated before surgery. In addition, the patient showed optimal oral hygiene. It was also an explicit wish of the patient that no implantological treatment be carried out in the lower jaw (Figs. 11.2, 11.3, 11.4, 11.5, and 11.6).

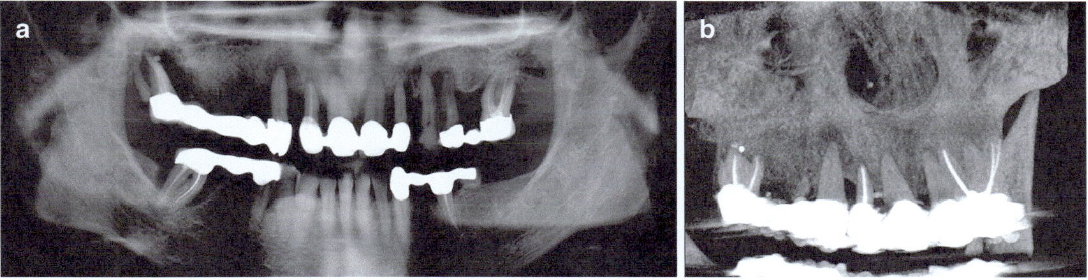

Fig. 11.2 (**a**, **b**) Due to the attachment loss of the teeth in the maxilla, and after intensive discussion and planning with the patient, it was decided to extract the teeth in the upper jaw. (© Andreas Schlegel 2021. All Rights Reserved)

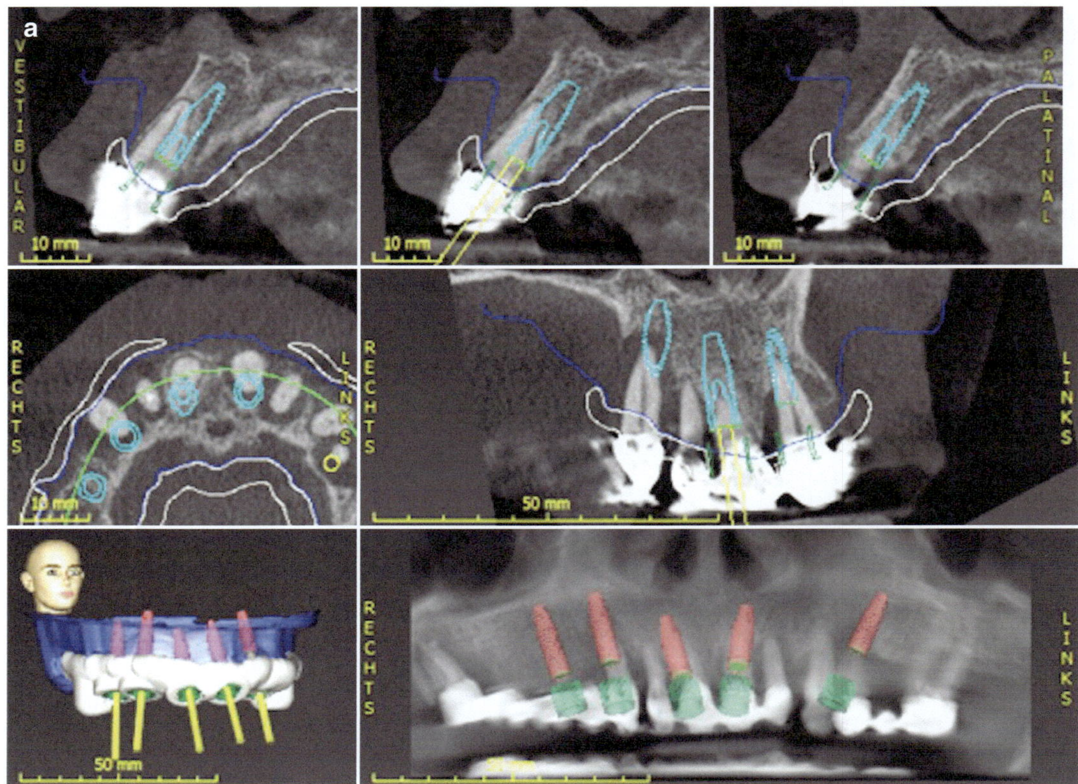

Fig. 11.3 (**a–c**) In this case, two tooth-borne templates were used. The first template was supported on a few anterior teeth and the second template on implant pins in the posterior region (**c**). (© Andreas Schlegel 2021. All Rights Reserved)

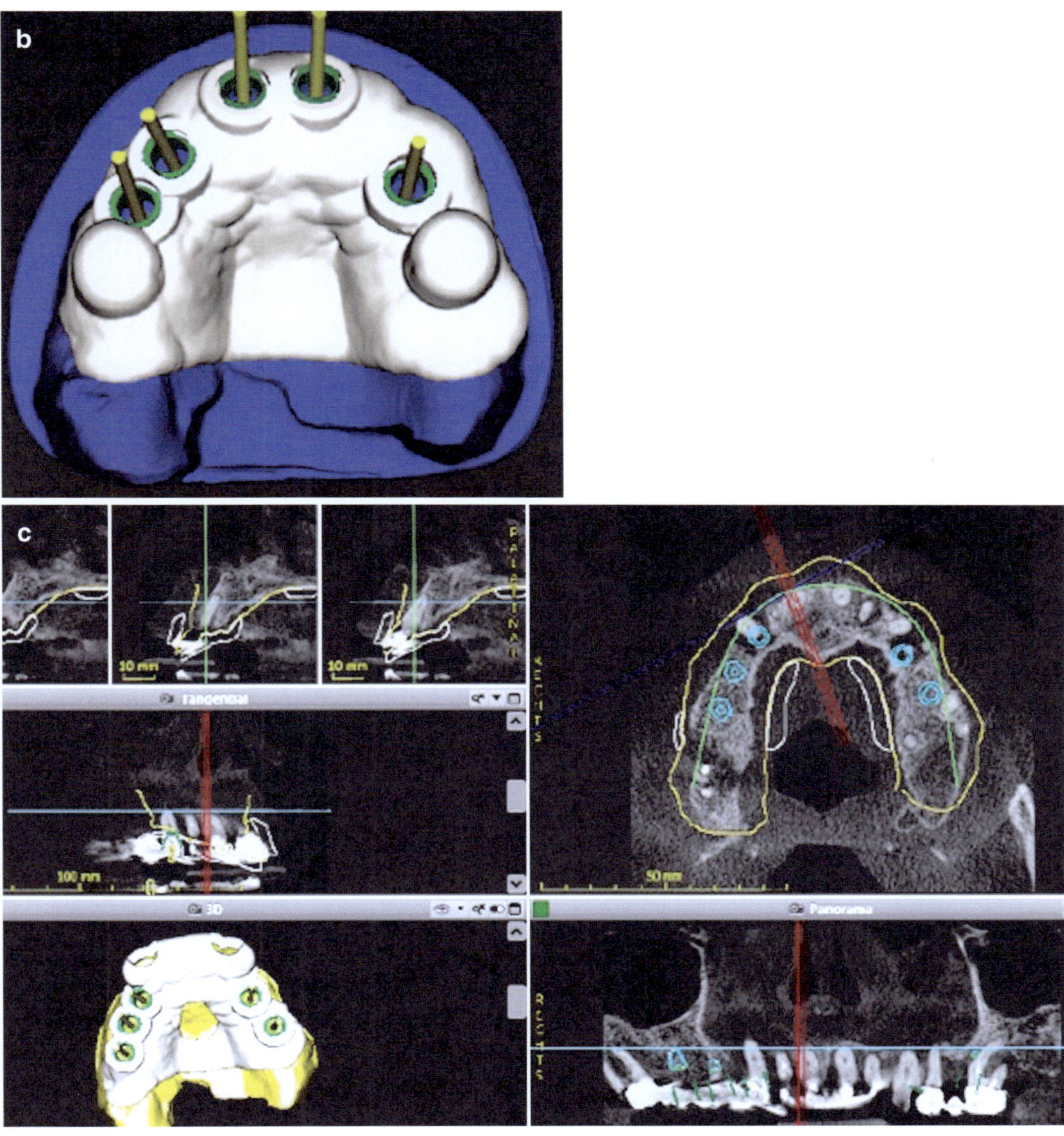

Fig. 11.3 (continued)

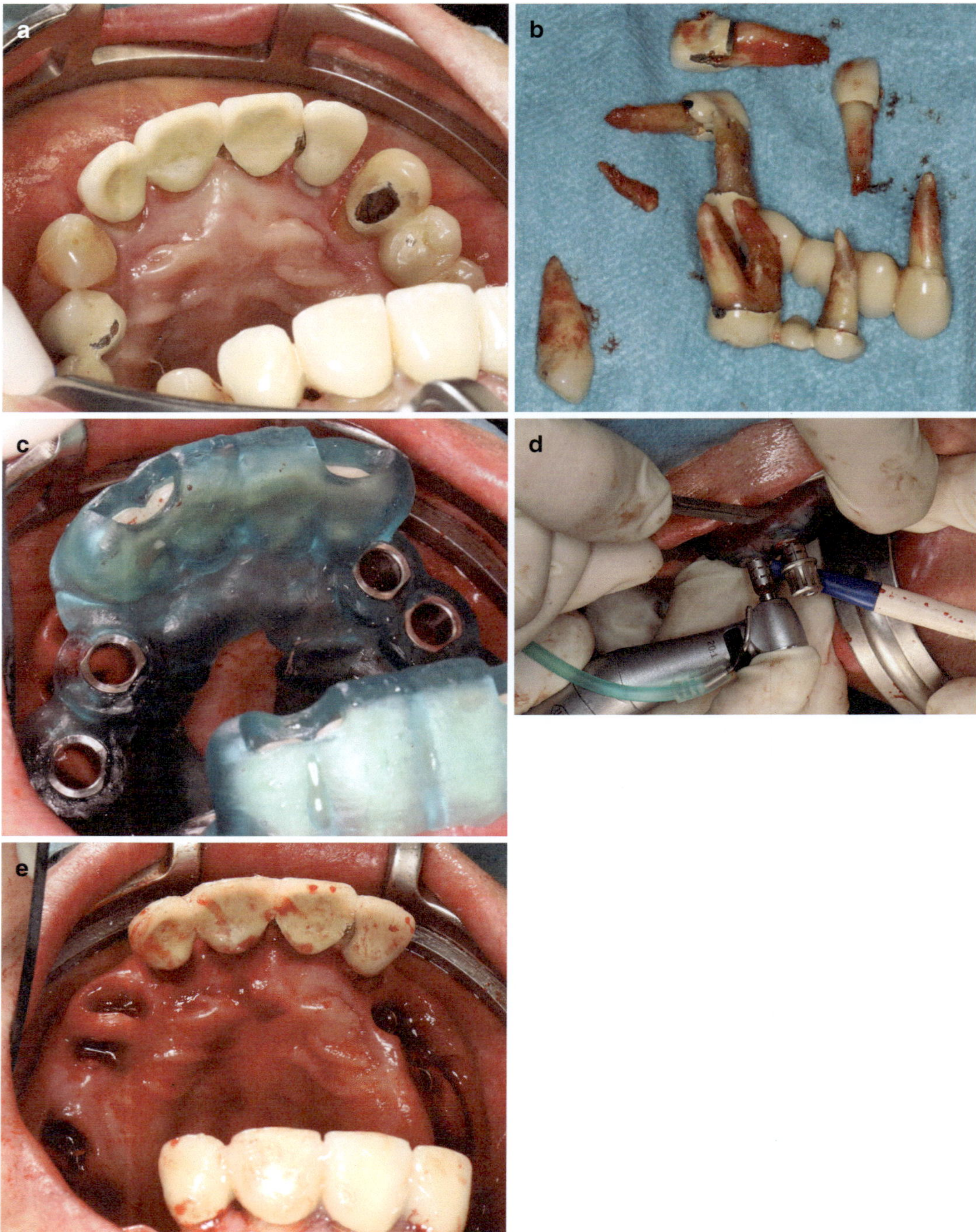

Fig. 11.4 (**a–e**) The first splint, which was tooth-borne on the incisors, is shown. After the first implant placement in the posterior region, the splints were changed. (© Andreas Schlegel 2021. All Rights Reserved)

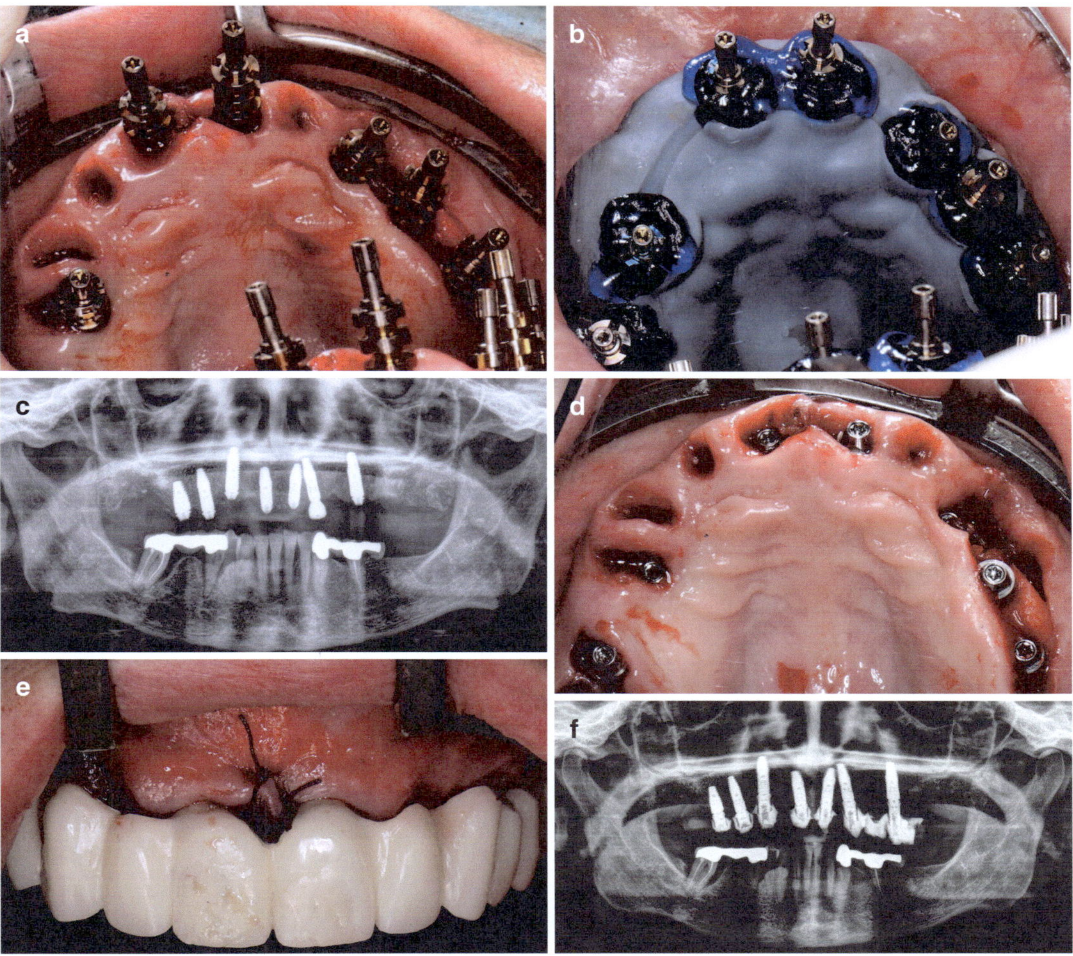

Fig. 11.5 (**a–f**) After all the implants had been inserted (good stability is very important), the intraoperative implant impression was taken. The prefabricated full-arch denture was finally inserted after bonding the individual connection elements. (© Andreas Schlegel 2021. All Rights Reserved)

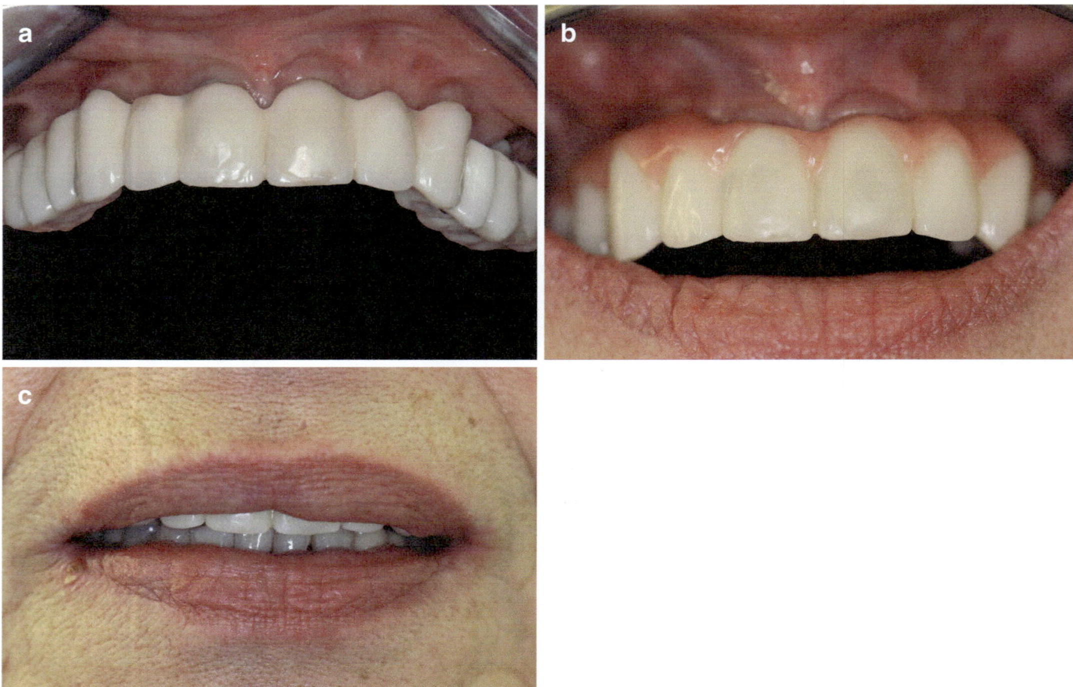

Fig. 11.6 (**a–c**) After 3 months, the final fixed denture could be inserted. (© Andreas Schlegel 2021. All Rights Reserved)

References

1. Gallucci GO, Benic GI, Eckert SE, Papaspyridakos P, Schimmel M, Schrott A, Weber HP. Consensus statements and clinical recommendations for implant loading protocols. Int J Oral Maxillofac Implants. 2014;29(Suppl):287–90.
2. Buser D, Chappuis V, Belser UC, Chen S. Implant placement post extraction in esthetic single tooth sites: when immediate, when early, when late? Periodontology. 2017;2000(73):84–102.
3. Al YF, Camenisch B, Al-Sabbagh M. Is digital guided implant surgery accurate and reliable? Dent Clin N Am. 2019;63:381–97.
4. Degidi M, Piattelli A. Comparative analysis study of 702 dental implants subjected to immediate functional loading and immediate nonfunctional loading to traditional healing periods with a follow-up of up to 24 months. Int J Oral Maxillofac Implants. 2005;20:99–107.
5. Degidi M, Piattelli A. Immediate functional and non-functional loading of dental implants: a 2- to 60-month follow-up study of 646 titanium implants. J Periodontol. 2003;74:225–41.
6. Baruffaldi A, Poli PP, Baruffaldi A, Giberti L, Pigozzo M, Maiorana C. Computer-aided flapless implant surgery and immediate loading. A technical note. Oral Maxillofac Surg. 2016;20:313–9.
7. D'haese J, Ackhurst J, Wismeijer D, De Bruyn H, Tahmaseb A. Current state of the art of computer-guided implant surgery. Periodontology. 2017;2000(73):121–33.
8. Lages FS, Douglas-De Oliveira DW, Costa FO. Relationship between implant stability measurements obtained by insertion torque and resonance frequency analysis: a systematic review. Clin Implant Dent Relat Res. 2018;20:26–33.

Digital Workflow After Implant Placement: Clinical Cases

12.1 Case I: With Flap

In addition to full-guided planning before surgery, digital processes can also be used directly after implant placement. In this approach, the implant position is recorded directly after the insertion of the implant body via scan bodies. Afterward, the digital data can be sent to the referring colleagues for immediate restoration, for example, to obtain long-term temporaries in the shortest possible time. In this case, 3 zirconia implants were inserted in regions 11, 21, and 24 (Figs. 12.1, 12.2, 12.3, 12.4, 12.5, 12.6, 12.7, 12.8, and 12.9). When opting for immediate restoration, we suggest avoiding occlusal loading as much as possible and eliminating occlusal contact points. The long-term temporaries could be inserted on the day of surgery using screw fixation. The soft tissue was already conditioned from the time of implant placement. Finally, after 3 months, the final crowns were inserted.

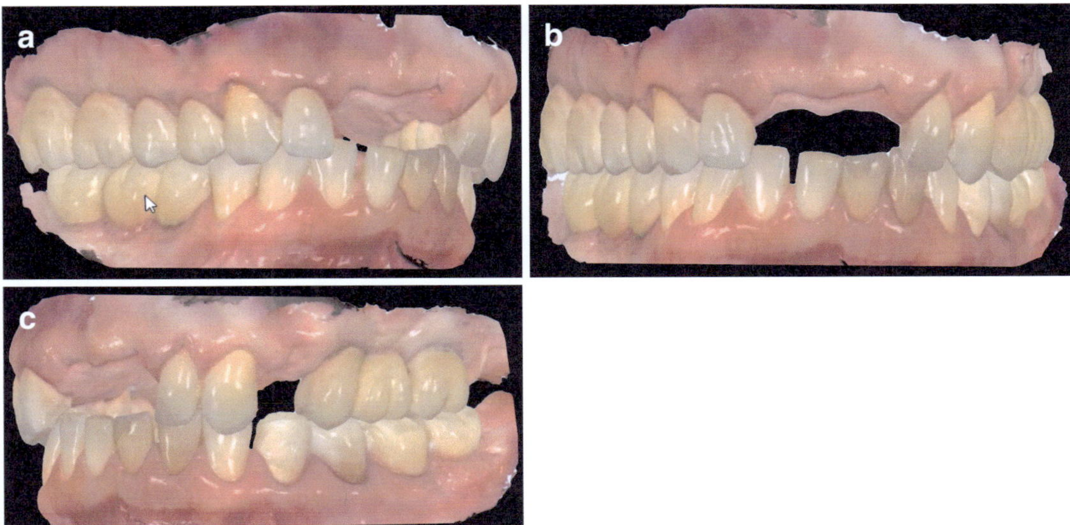

Fig. 12.1 (**a–c**) Preoperative intraoral scan images of the maxilla and mandible in habitual occlusion. (© Heinz Kniha 2021. All Rights Reserved)

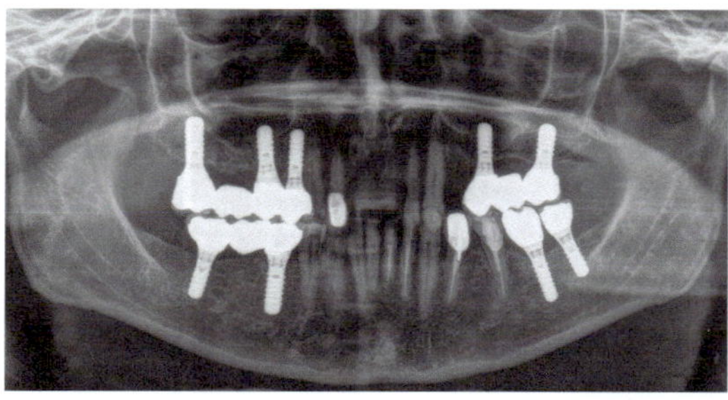

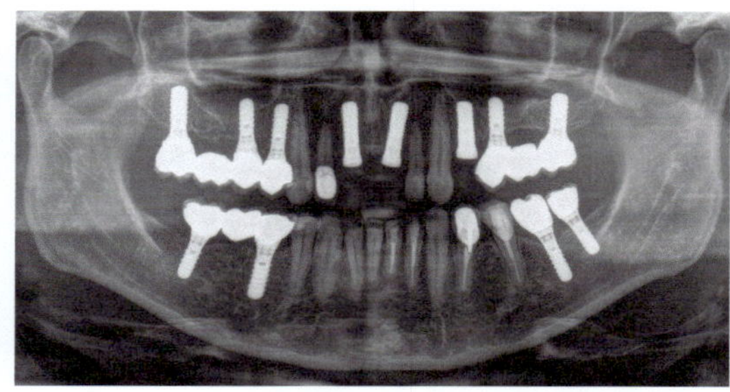

Fig. 12.2 Radiological initial situation with missing teeth in regions 11, 21, and 24. (© Heinz Kniha 2021. All Rights Reserved)

Fig. 12.3 Postoperative radiological control image after the implant placement of 3 zirconium dioxide implants in regions 11, 21, and 24. (© Heinz Kniha 2021. All Rights Reserved)

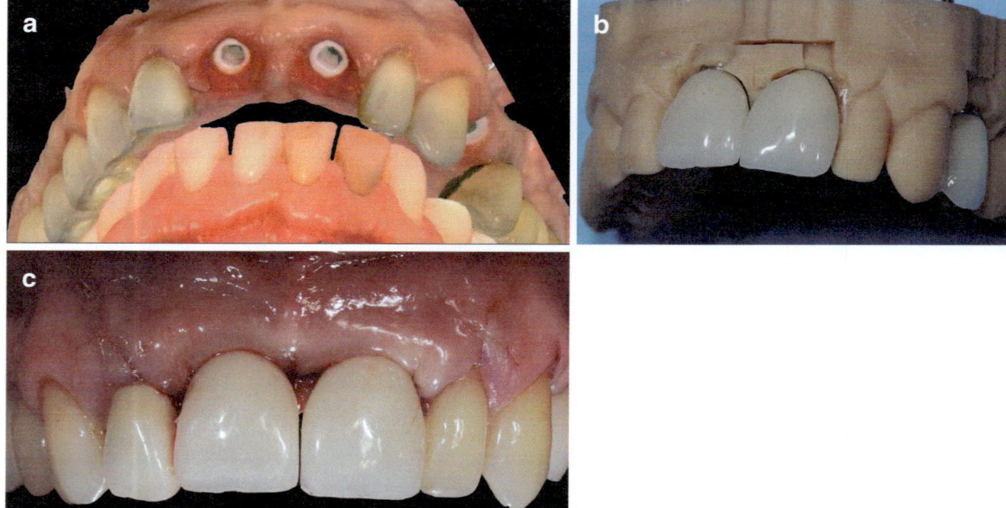

Fig. 12.4 (**a–c**) During surgery, the implant positions were scanned. Immediate prosthetic restoration was performed without immediate occlusal loading of the implants in regions 11, 21, and 24 after 4 h. ((**a, c**) © Heinz Kniha 2021. All Rights Reserved except (**b**) © Thomas Lassen)

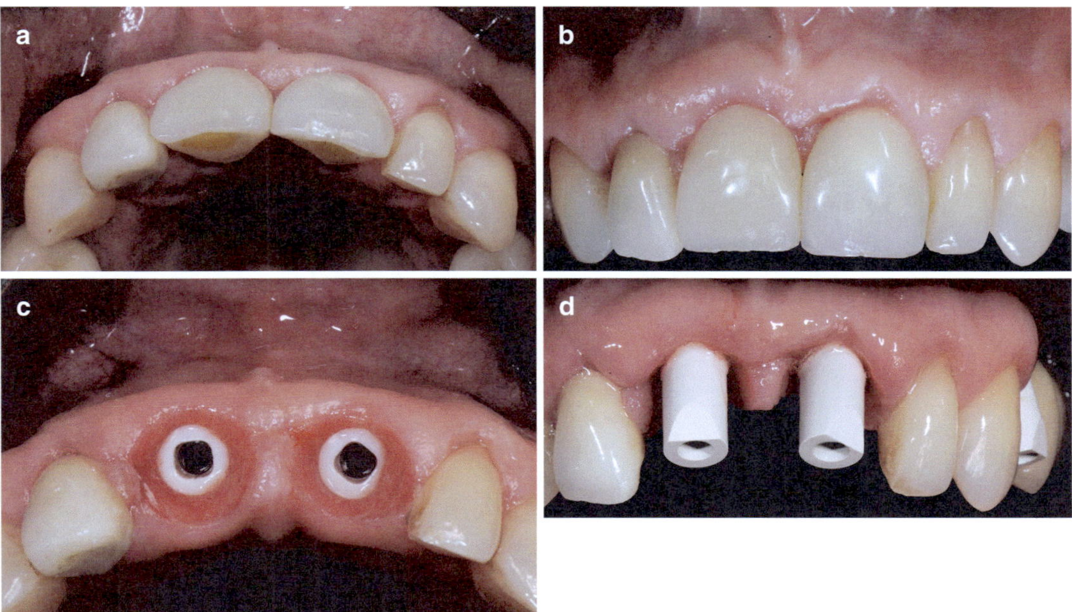

Fig. 12.5 (**a–d**) After wearing the long-term temporary crowns for 3 months, digital impressions for the final crowns were taken. At this follow-up appointment, the soft tissue was pale and inflammation-free. (© Heinz Kniha 2021. All Rights Reserved)

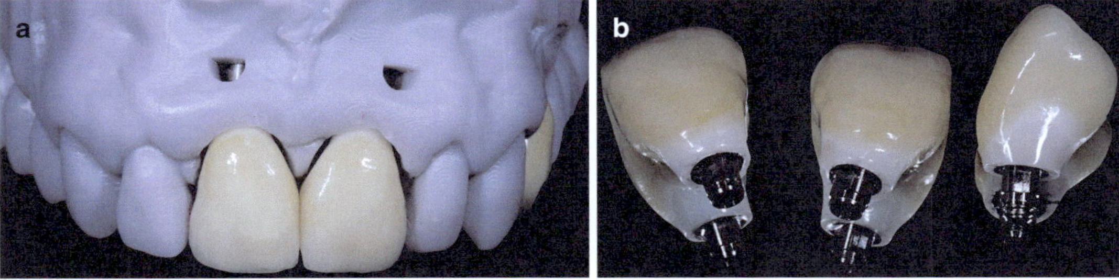

Fig. 12.6 (**a, b**) The definitive crowns were fabricated using the digital impressions and were retained with screws. (© Thomas Lassen)

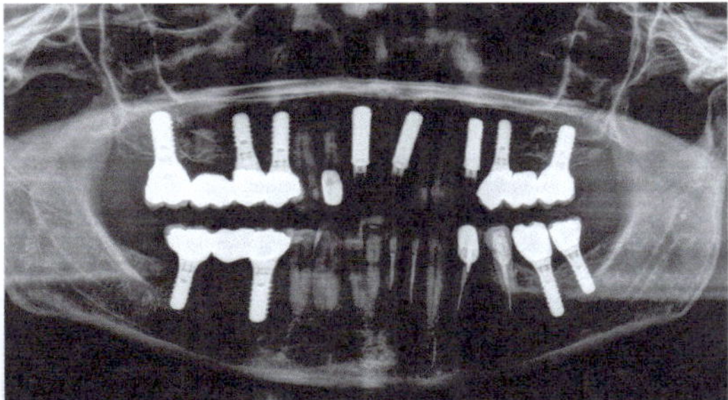

Fig. 12.7 Radiologic imaging showed that the peri-implant crestal bone remained stable after 3 months of follow-up. (© Heinz Kniha 2021. All Rights Reserved)

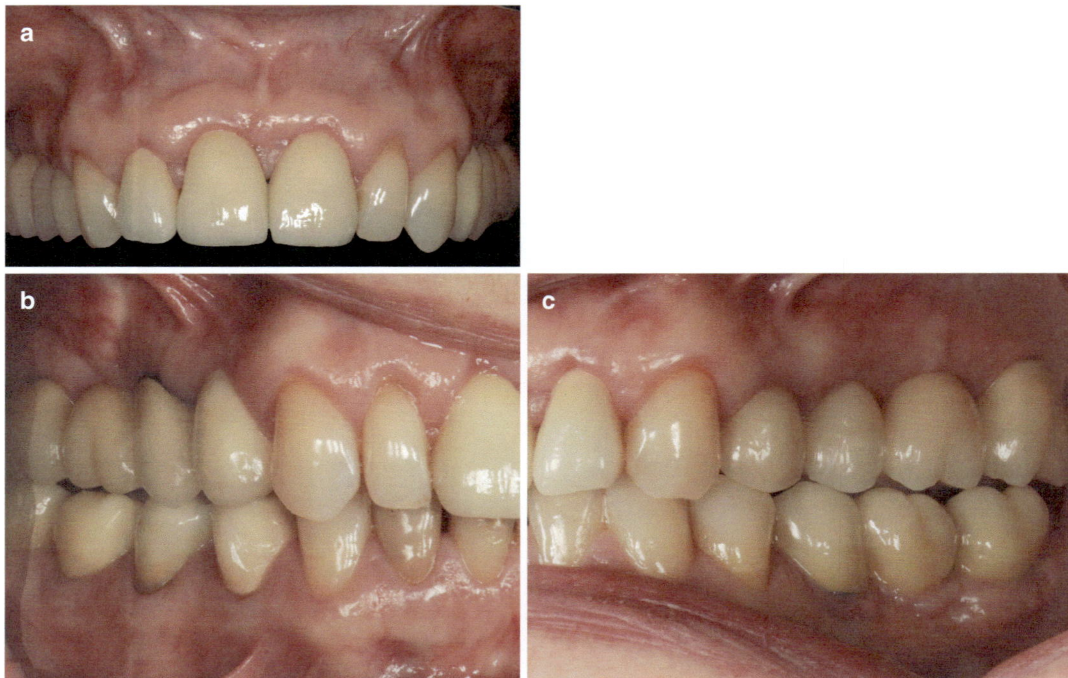

Fig. 12.8 (**a–c**) Four weeks after the placement of the final crowns, there was a further harmonization of the soft tissues and a filling of the interdental papillae. (© Heinz Kniha 2021. All Rights Reserved)

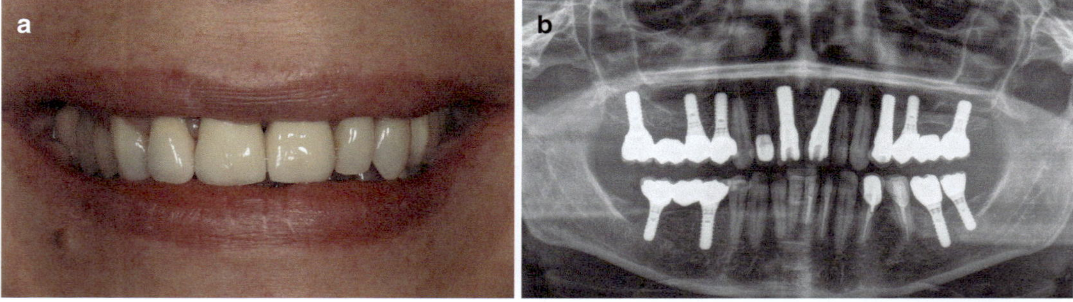

Fig. 12.9 (**a, b**) These images show, on the one hand, the radiological situation after screwing the crowns and, on the other hand, the clinical smile line in the esthetic zone. (© Heinz Kniha 2021. All Rights Reserved)

12.2   Case II: Flapless

In this case, tooth 22 showed periapical inflammation and tooth mobility (Fig. 12.10). After root removal and a 3-month healing period, a delayed zirconia implant was placed (Figs. 12.11 and 12.12). With this patient, no immediate restoration was planned and a zirconia healing cap was inserted. After the healing phase, intraoral scans were performed for the final crown fabrication. In Fig. 12.13, the digital workflow is shown (Figs. 12.14, 12.15, and 12.16).

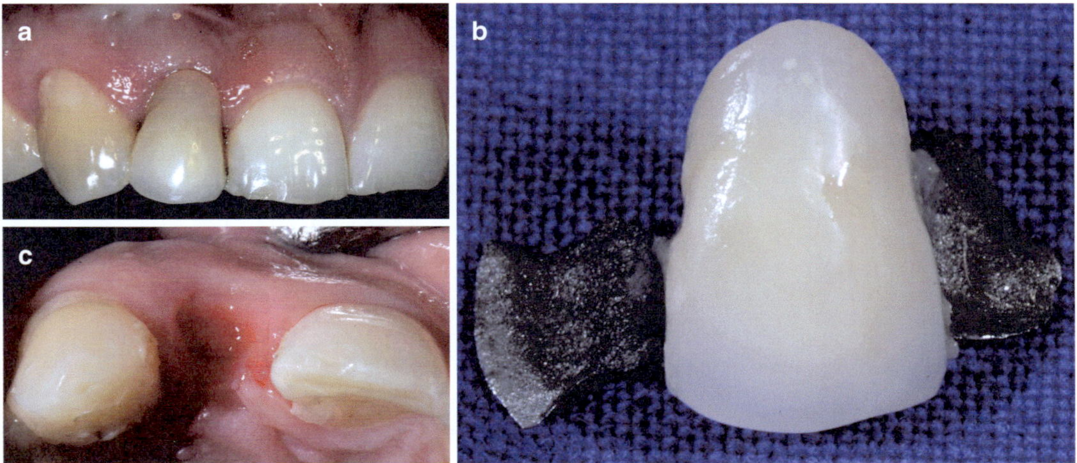

Fig. 12.10 (a–c) In this case, the gap was provisionally restored with an adhesive bridge. (© Heinz Kniha 2021. All Rights Reserved)

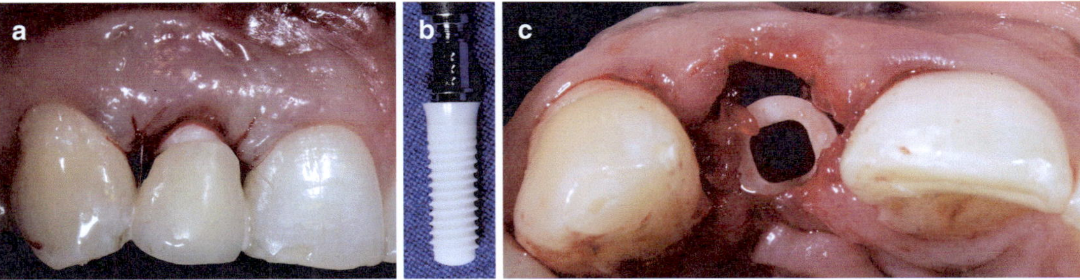

Fig. 12.11 (a–c) The root extraction was followed by the immediate placement of a zirconia implant. Healing took place transgingivally with a zirconia healing cap. (© Heinz Kniha 2021. All Rights Reserved)

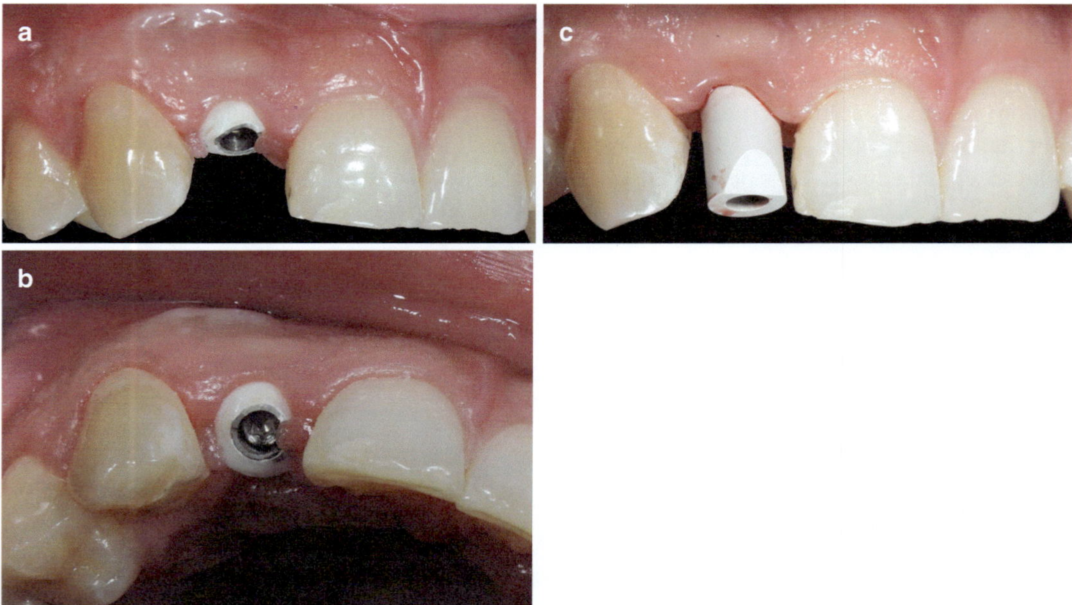

Fig. 12.12 (**a–c**) After a 3-month unloaded healing phase, the implant presented successful integration, and the impressions of the jaws were taken using intraoral scans and a scan body. (© Heinz Kniha 2021. All Rights Reserved)

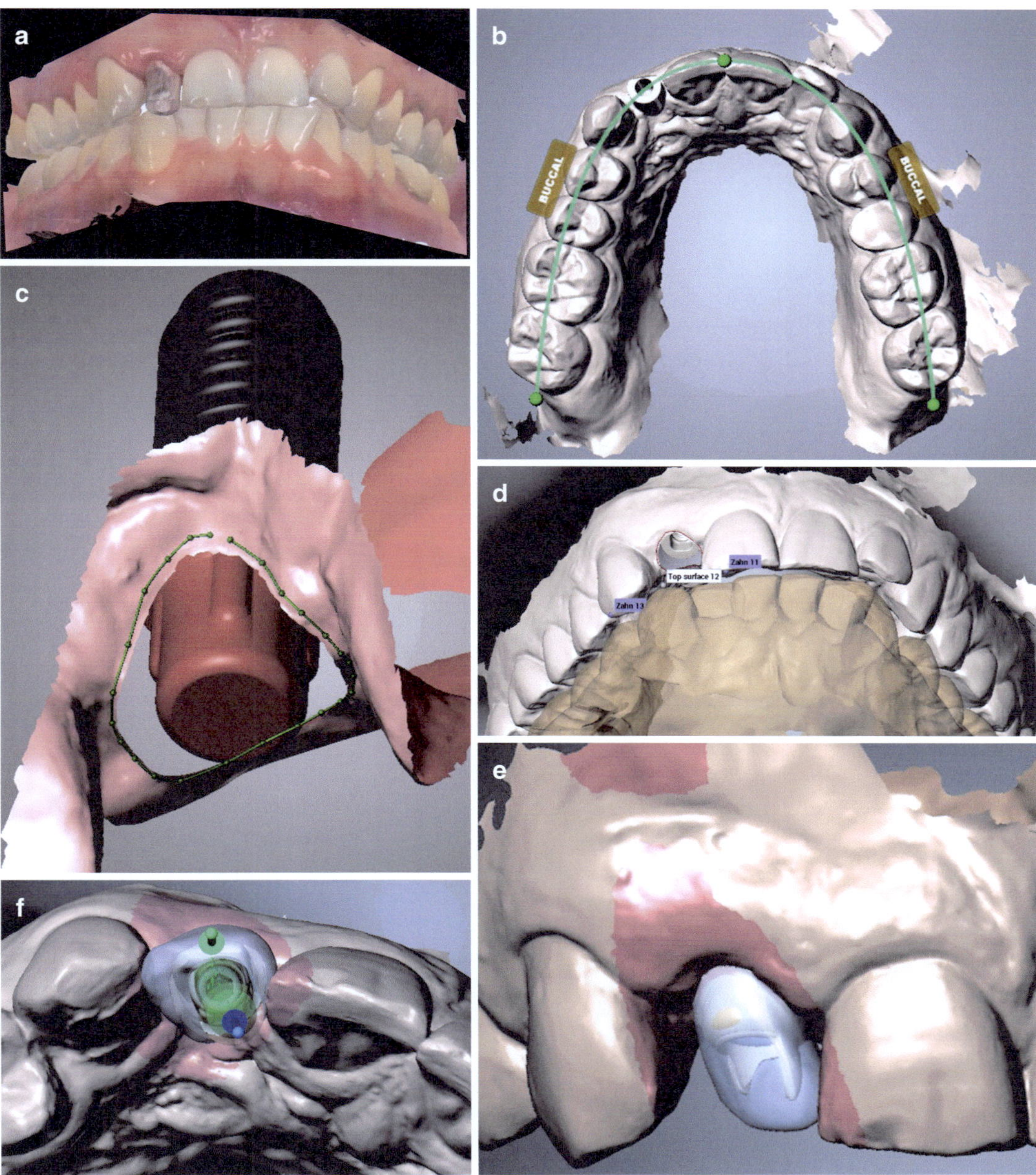

Fig. 12.13 (**a–f**) The digital data set could then be transmitted to the dental technician. In the laboratory, the gingiva margin was marked in a software program, and the insertion direction was determined. ((**a**) © Heinz Kniha 2021. All Rights Reserved except (**b–f**) © Thomas Lassen)

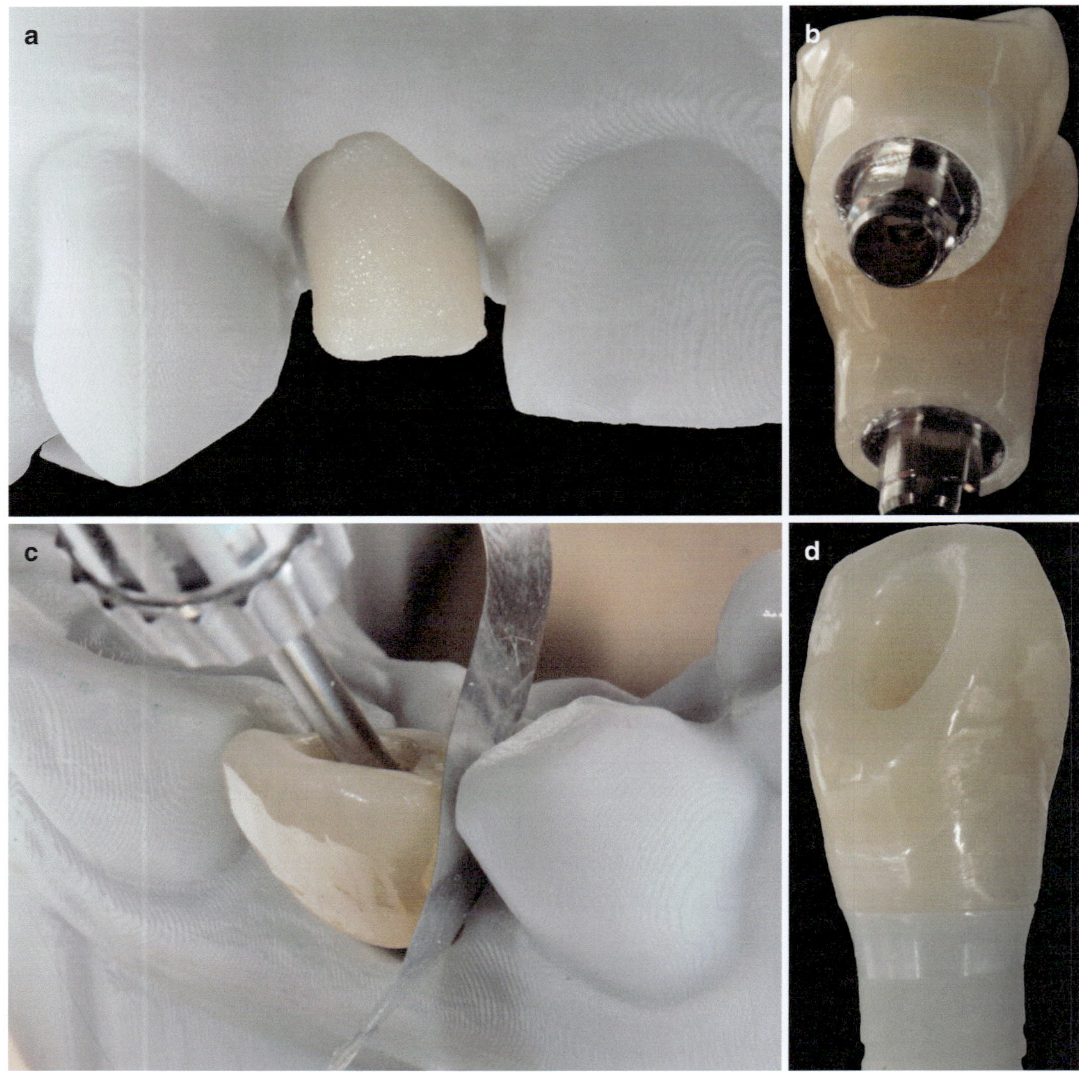

Fig. 12.14 (**a–d**) Finally, the crown was fabricated using a bonded titanium base and was subsequently fixed using a screw. (© Thomas Lassen)

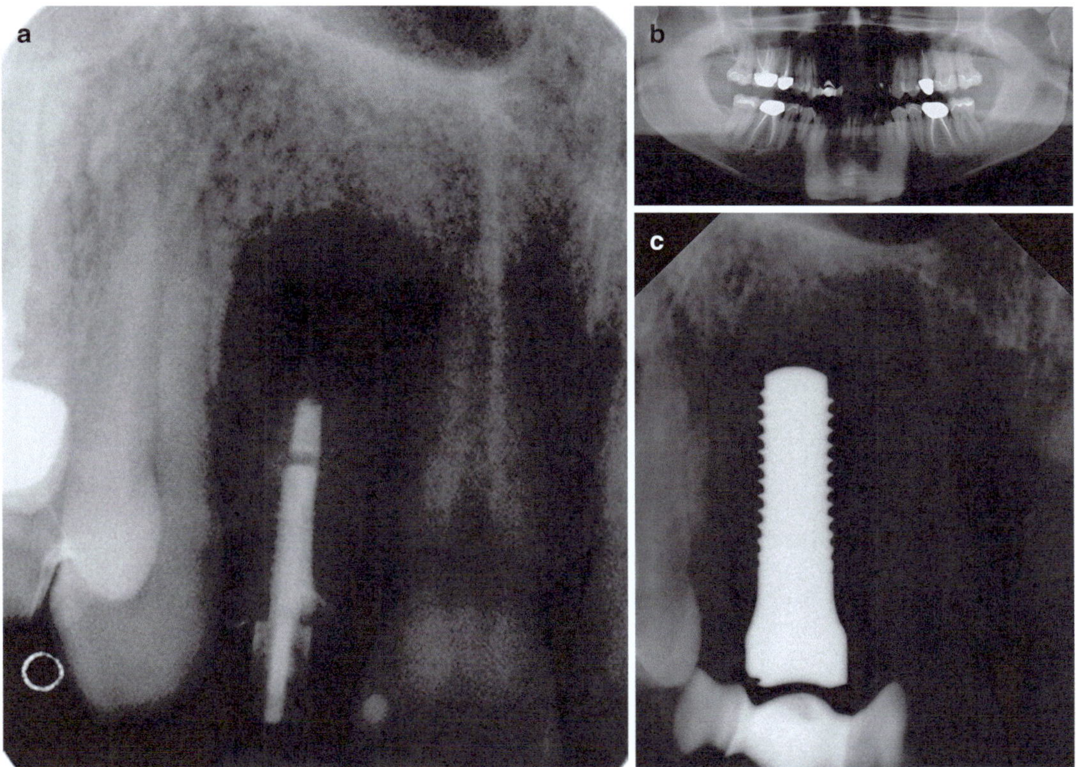

Fig. 12.15 (**a–c**) The radiographic course over time is presented and (**a**) was recorded before the tooth extraction and (**b**) after the healing phase of 3 months. The X-ray in (**c**) was recorded directly after the implant placement. (© Heinz Kniha 2021. All Rights Reserved)

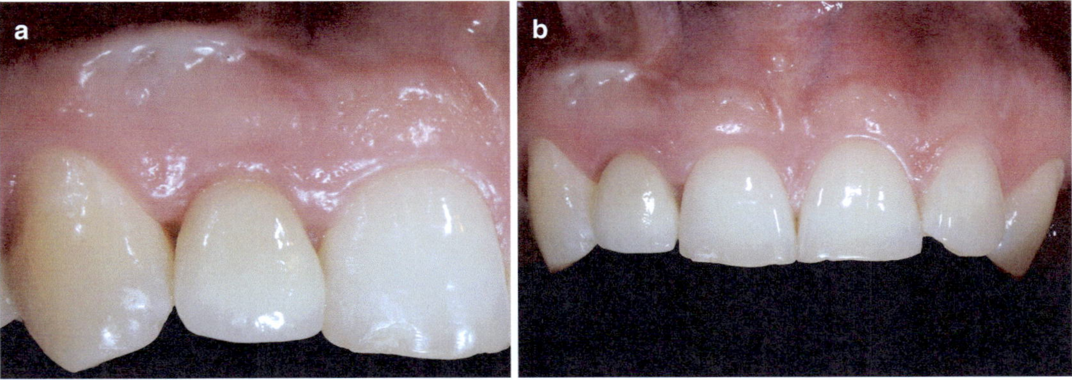

Fig. 12.16 (**a, b**) In both figures, the clinical follow-up 4 weeks after crown placement is presented. Papillary fill improved after crown placement. (© Heinz Kniha 2021. All Rights Reserved)

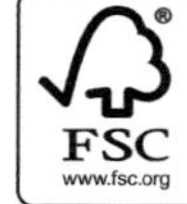

MIX
Papier aus verantwortungsvollen Quellen
Paper from responsible sources
FSC® C105338

If you have any concerns about our products,
you can contact us on
ProductSafety@springernature.com

In case Publisher is established outside the EU,
the EU authorized representative is:
Springer Nature Customer Service Center GmbH
Europaplatz 3, 69115 Heidelberg, Germany

Printed by Libri Plureos GmbH
in Hamburg, Germany